Your Mouth: Oral Care for All Ages

Chilton's Better Health Series

FRANK E. TAYLOR, EDITOR

Your Skin: Its Problems and Care
by Setrag A. Zacarian, M.D.
Your Mouth: Oral Care for All Ages
by Nguyen Thanh Nguyen, D.D.S., with Patty de Roulf

YOUR MOUTH
Oral Care for All Ages

NGUYEN THANH NGUYEN, D.D.S.
with PATTY DE ROULF

A Frank E. Taylor Book

CHILTON BOOK COMPANY
RADNOR, PENNSYLVANIA

Published in Radnor, Pennsylvania, by Chilton Book Company
and simultaneously in Don Mills, Ontario, Canada,
by Thomas Nelson & Sons, Ltd.
Manufactured in the United States of America
Design by Adrianne Onderdonk Dudden

Library of Congress Cataloging in Publication Data

Nguyen Thanh Nguyen
Your mouth.

(Chilton's better health series)
"a Frank E. Taylor book"

Includes index.
1.Dentistry—Popular works. 2.Teeth—Care and hygiene. I.DeRoulf, Patty, joint author. II.Title.
RK61.N48 617.6 78-7180
ISBN 0-8019-6667-1

CHILTON'S BETTER HEALTH SERIES
Frank E. Taylor, Editor

1 2 3 4 5 6 7 8 9 0 7 6 5 4 3 2 1 0 9

To our families

CONTENTS

ACKNOWLEDGMENTS

The authors would like to express their appreciation to Dr. James P. Voight, Department of Dental Health Education at the University of Pennsylvania School of Dental Medicine, and to Dr. Anthony G. Roeder, past president of the American Society for Preventive Dentistry, for their review and suggestions in the preparation of this manuscript. Special thanks go to Susan Quan for her outstanding illustrations. We are greatly indebted to Mary E. Herrera for her assistance in putting the book together. Also, we are particularly grateful to Kathryn Conover for her splendid editing. We would have liked to acknowledge here every person who has contributed, in even a small way, to this book. They are too numerous to list.

Finally, I (N.T.N.) want to thank my friend and teacher, Werner Erhard, founder of est, for all the satisfaction and value I have gotten from our association. Werner showed me how to get my life filled with the joy of service, participation and contribution, how to effortlessly expand my commitment to the quality of others' lives.

Your Mouth: Oral Care for All Ages

With best wishes for
an excellent oral health
to Lamon Harkness
Jewett

Sincerely
N Nguyen
San Francisco May 30th 1979

INTRODUCTION

In this age of great scientific advances, every man, woman and child could have beautiful, healthy teeth and gums. There is no longer a reason to dread the dentist's drill, because dentistry has become truly painless. There is no reason to fear extractions, because teeth can be saved. There is no reason to have cavities or irritated gums, because preventive dentistry can wipe out tooth decay and gum problems.

But all the dentists in the world cannot save your teeth without your cooperation. They are your teeth and *you have more control over your teeth than over any other part of your body.*

Most of us were born with perfect teeth. But what happened as the years went by? A cavity here, a cavity there, bleeding gums, a cap, an abscess, an extraction. Hours spent in the dental chair, thousands of dollars spent in dental fees.

Only 2 percent of the American population somehow escapes dental woes. For the rest of us, mouth problems are more common than the common cold. Even worse, they start at a very early age. Fifty percent of our 2-year-olds already have cavities, and 24 out of 25 6-year-olds suffer dental trouble in one form or another. Considering all ages, some 90 million of us have had at least 18 out of 32 teeth extracted, filled or left to decay. And one-eighth of the population is toothless!

The problem is as old as time. Excavated skulls of cavemen show an occasional missing tooth and scientists believe that, whenever an ancestor had a toothache, a friend obligingly knocked it out with a stone. The Egyptians were perhaps the first to get into dentistry. They regarded it as a branch of medicine and were clever at fashioning false teeth from gold or ivory, then neatly wiring them in place.

It was the ancient Hindus who developed some of the earliest real dental equipment. They drilled teeth and filled the holes with gold or glittering jewels if the patient was affluent. Hindus also carried toothpicks made from aromatic wood and, as early as 2700 BC, the Chinese were using acupuncture to cure toothaches.

Dentistry in Europe remained primitive until the Middle Ages. Instruments were crude. Fillings were made of resins, gums, plaster and waxes. No one understood the process of decay, nor were there any techniques for removing decay from a tooth.

Much later, soft gold fillings came into use. Tiny pieces of gold were packed into a cavity in a procedure that required hours of work. All too often, the filling soon crumbled and fell out. It wasn't until early in the nineteenth century that a French dentist, M. Taveau, filed down some silver coins, mixed the silver powder with mercury, and came up with the first amalgam fillings. Unfortunately, an unfounded fear that the mercury in the filling could harm a patient prevented amalgam from being fully accepted until 1895. Today, amalgam fillings are used extensively.

General anesthesia was accepted by the medical profession in 1844, but it was another 60 years before local anesthesia came on the scene. Both were godsends. Around 1890, the original hand-cranked dental drill was replaced by a foot-pedal drill. Twenty years later, x-ray machines became generally available. Then came cast-gold inlays, porcelain crowns, orthodontics, endodontics, periodontics and, finally, the first widespread public awareness of preventive dentistry.

We have come a long way. Today America has 130,000 well-trained dentists, the highest dental standards in the world, and the most modern equipment. Then why must we spend nearly 9 billion dollars annually for dental work, much of it avoidable, on top of more than half a billion dollars we pay for toothpaste and toothbrushes?

Ignorance could be the answer. Sadly, most of us know almost nothing about our teeth and gums, nor do we know how to care for them properly. Few of us yet realize that dental decay and periodontal disease are 100 percent preventable through plaque eradication, home and office fluoride therapy, and proper nutrition. Believing this and transforming our behavior to take advantage of the latest concepts of dentistry can mean freedom from tooth decay and periodontal disease.

This book was written to show how this freedom can be achieved. As a first step, you should become familiar with your teeth and gums, able to recognize dental problems, know what your dentist can do for you and, especially, what you can do for yourself.

1 YOUR TEETH
Things you never knew about them

Your teeth are vital, living tissues and deserve as much of your consideration and time in caring for them as your face, your hair, or any other part of your body.

Why do we need healthy teeth? For three good reasons: To chew. To speak. To look attractive. The key to a successful oral hygiene program is believing that you can save your teeth. You have the choice of excellent dental health over poor dental health and the problems that go with it. Knowledge alone won't do the job: you must perform daily, diligent home oral care, because the dentist cannot make up for years of neglect in a one-hour appointment. Remember that dental disease is more easily prevented than cured and that you—and only you—are in control of your mouth. If you conscientiously do your part, you'll thank yourself every day of your life.

The human mouth is a collection of highly sensitive organs associated with love, hate, affection, cruelty and frustration. If teeth and gums are in optimal health, they can contribute to maintaining proper body balance. Good dental health not only facilitates efficient digestion of food, but can impart warmth, confidence and friendliness. Good mouth hygiene prevents diseased teeth and gums and offensive odors, unspoken conditions for social acceptance. We all want to be healthy, loved and successful in life. Accomplishing these goals includes maintenance of good dental health, for it plays an important role in physical and emotional well being. First, let's understand and appreciate the assets we have in healthy teeth.

Primary Teeth

By the time you were born, you had a full set of twenty teeth. As you grew, these teeth were also developing, in fact pressing against the bones in your jaws. One day a little white speck of enamel peeked through your gum. This first tooth was undoubtedly a lower middle front tooth, and it erupted when you were 5 or 6 months old. Soon, another front tooth erupted, probably next to the first one. A month or so later, two more teeth appeared to either side of the first ones. The same procedure occurred shortly afterward in the upper jaw, and new teeth continued to appear until the final second molar erupted at about the age of 2 years. You now had twenty baby teeth or milk teeth, properly called *primary* or *deciduous teeth.* The accompanying illustration shows the relationships and positions of the primary teeth, along with their code letters and correct names.

Primary teeth don't last, of course. It takes 2 or 3 years for them to become completely formed; then, before you know it, they begin to loosen up and make way for permanent teeth in a process called *exfoliation.* Incisors are the first to go, falling out quite easily at the age of 6 to 8 years. The first molar tends to get somewhat wobbly when a child is about 8 or 9. At approximately 11 years, the second molars and the cuspids are exfoliated.

Permanent Teeth

Your first permanent molars were already beginning to grow the day you were born. While primary teeth were still erupting,

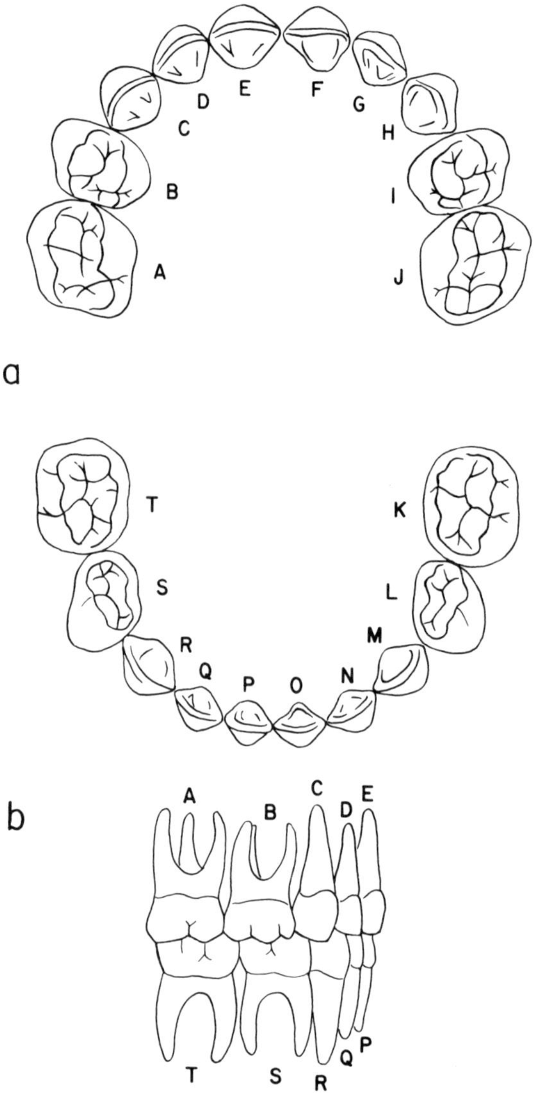
A B C D E F G H I J
a
T S R Q P O N M L K
b
A B C D E
T S R Q P

other tooth buds were forming below the gumline. The buds developed quietly until about the age of 6. Then came a dynamic change, as the buds forced themselves into position. The buds grew into permanent teeth that pressed against the roots of the primary teeth, finally pushing so hard that the roots of the primary teeth dissolved. Only the crowns of the deciduous teeth were left. Attached loosely to gum tissue, the hollow crowns were easily shed.

Even before one of your primary teeth could be wiggled with a finger, your first permanent tooth was sprouting. That tooth, often called the 6-year molar because it appears at about age 6, technically is known as the first molar. There are four of them—upper and lower left and upper and lower right—always the sixth tooth counting from the midline. These first molars do not replace primary teeth and are supposed to last the rest of your life.

These four first molars determine the position of all other permanent teeth and are known as the cornerstones of the dental arches. So if you are a parent, a word of warning: a child's 6-year molar is often mistaken for another baby tooth and sometimes neglected or even extracted. Its rate of decay early in life is exceedingly high; if it is lost, the whole arch of teeth can become poorly balanced and a child's bite will suffer.

At approximately 5 years of age, spaces often appear between the teeth. The reason is that the jaws are growing. They must

Primary teeth. (a) The primary arch; key identifies teeth with corresponding alphabet letters, followed by approximate eruption date. (b) Primary teeth in occlusion.

A—UR second molar, 24 to 26 months
B—UR first molar, 14 to 16 months
C—UR cuspid, 18 to 20 months
D—UR lateral incisor, 9 to 11 months
E—UR central incisor, 7 to 9 months
F—UL central incisor, 7 to 9 months
G—UL lateral incisor, 9 to 11 months
H—UL cuspid, 18 to 20 months
I—UL first molar, 14 to 16 months
J—UL second molar, 24 to 26 months
K—LL second molar, 20 to 22 months
L—LL first molar, 12 to 14 months
M—LL cuspid, 16 to 18 months
N—LL lateral incisor, 7 to 9 months
O—LL central incisor, 6 to 8 months
P—LR central incisor, 6 to 8 months
Q—LR lateral incisor, 7 to 9 months
R—LR cuspid, 16 to 18 months
S—LR first molar, 12 to 14 months
T—LR second molar, 20 to 22 months

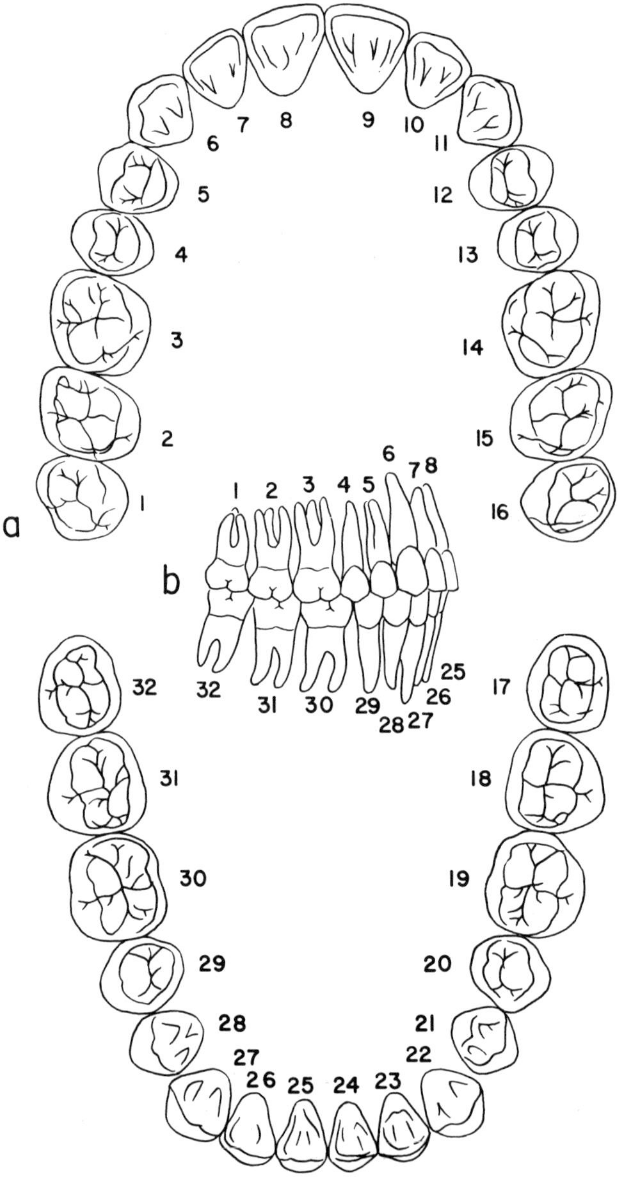
a
1
2
3
4
5
6
7
8
9
10
11
12
13
14
15
16
17
18
19
20
21
22
23
24
25
26
27
28
29
30
31
32
b
1
2
3
4
5
6
7
8
32
31
30
29
28
27
26
25

get larger, because permanent teeth are going to be a lot bigger than primary teeth. Upper and lower jaws grow in both a forward and a backward direction. After the first molars, the permanent central incisors appear, followed by lateral incisors, premolars, cuspids and second molars. The premolars usually erupt at 10 to 11½ years of age, in the place occupied by the primary molars. Second molars erupt at about the age of 12 and, finally, the third molars (wisdom teeth) may or may not show up between the ages of 17 and 21. If all teeth come in, you should have thirty-two, as shown in the diagram with code numbers and proper names. When your permanent teeth first appear, they are by no means fully formed and must still complete their calcification.

The incisors, central and lateral, are chisel-shaped and have sharp edges to cut and chop up food. The cuspid is apt to be pointed and is often called a canine, because it is shaped like a dog's tooth. It serves to grasp and tear at food. Primary molars, both first and second, have a broad, flat surface and their job is to grind food so that it may be easily swallowed.

Permanent teeth. (a) The permanent arch; key identifies each tooth by corresponding number, followed by approximate eruption date. (b) Permanent teeth in occlusion.

1—UR third molar, 17 to 21 years
2—UR second molar, 12 to 13 years
3—UR first molar, 6 to 7 years
4—UR second bicuspid, 10 to 12 years
5—UR first bicuspid, 10 to 11 years
6—UR cuspid, 11 to 12 years
7—UR lateral incisor, 8 to 9 years
8—UR central incisor, 7 to 8 years
9—UL central incisor, 7 to 8 years
10—UL lateral incisor, 8 to 9 years
11—UL cuspid, 11 to 12 years
12—UL first bicuspid, 10 to 11 years
13—UL second bicuspid, 10 to 12 years
14—UL first molar, 6 to 7 years
15—UL second molar, 12 to 13 years
16—UL third molar, 17 to 21 years
17—LL third molar, 17 to 21 years
18—LL second molar, 11 to 13 years
19—LL first molar, 6 to 7 years
20—LL second bicuspid, 11 to 12 years
21—LL first bicuspid, 10 to 12 years
22—LL cuspid, 9 to 10 years
23—LL lateral incisor, 7 to 8 years
24—LL central incisor, 6 to 7 years
25—LR central incisor, 6 to 7 years
26—LR lateral incisor, 7 to 8 years
27—LR cuspid, 9 to 10 years
28—LR first bicuspid, 10 to 12 years
29—LR second bicuspid, 11 to 12 years
30—LR first molar, 6 to 7 years
31—LR second molar, 11 to 13 years
32—LR third molar, 17 to 21 years

Tooth Structure

Every tooth has a crown, which is covered with hard white enamel, a root which is imbedded in the jawbone, and a cervix or neck, the section where the crown and root meet.

ENAMEL

Enamel is made up of rows of tiny rods that form a relatively smooth surface. This enamel is the hardest substance in a human body and is very resistant to friction and abrasion, but it does more than provide a chewing surface. It protects the inner dentin, which we shall describe shortly, insulating it against cold or heat. But there is one big problem with enamel: unlike other body tissues, it cannot repair or replace itself once it is worn down or injured.

ROOTS

The root forms the greater part of a tooth. Molars have two or three small roots fused together. There may even be as many as five or six in third molars. Most upper molars have three roots and lower molars have two roots. Other teeth have one root each, except for the first upper premolar, which usually is a "two-rooter."

CEMENTUM

Surrounding the roots of the teeth is a bonelike substance called cementum. It covers and protects the dentin from the bottom of the root to the cervix, where the enamel takes over.

Tiny fibers hold the roots in the jawbone, yet they are constantly separating from the cementum during eating or during eruption or injury. Just as constantly, the tiny fibers reattach themselves and, with the aid of new cementum being formed, everything continues to stick together. This miraculous process continues through the life of a tooth.

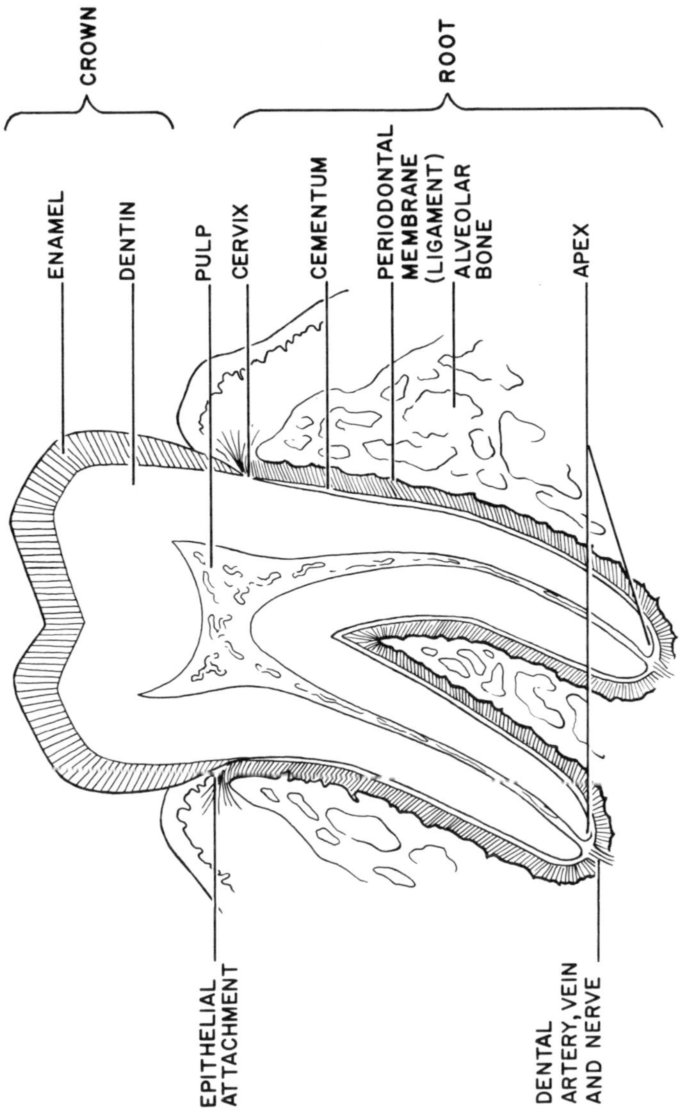

Tooth structure shown in cross section.

DENTIN

Dentin, the second hardest substance in your body, lies inside the crown and the root and forms the bulk of a tooth. Dentin is yellowish and contains numerous tiny canals through which it receives nourishment from the dental pulp. Dentin can do two things enamel can't: it can register pain and it can continue to reproduce itself as long as the pulp stays alive. Very important is the fact that dentin provides the elasticity needed while you chew. If that elasticity didn't exist, teeth would start to break after a few bites on a hard roll.

PULP

Pulp is the soft tissue which lies in the center of the root. It is a connective tissue containing blood vessels and nerve fibers. It is these nerve fibers that send pain signals to your brain when a cavity becomes larger and deeper. The pulp also nourishes the tooth, supplying fresh dentin day and night, especially during the formation of a new tooth or after injury to an old one. Pulp is literally the life of a tooth.

Everybody's teeth differ in color. The enamel surrounding the crown is a calcified material with a high mineral content but has no shade of its own. It merely reflects the shade of the dentin underneath. The thicker the dentin and the thinner the enamel, the darker the color of the tooth. The thicker the tooth enamel happens to be, the whiter and more translucent the tooth will appear.

Wisdom and Supernumerary Teeth

An individual may have as many as four impacted wisdom teeth (third molars), one buried in each corner of the jaws. Some people may have only three or two; occasionally there are none. That's why the wisdom tooth is called the disappearing tooth in civilized man. Quite probably, a third molar can't get out because the second molar is blocking its path, taking up the last available space. Jaws just don't grow long enough to accommodate third molars and they seem to be getting smaller with each generation.

There are good reasons for extracting impacted wisdom teeth, because they often lead to serious periodontal problems. They can aggravate the overcrowding of other teeth and may even become cystic (caused by inflammation of the follicular sac surrounding the crown of the impacted tooth) or cancerous. However, a deeply impacted wisdom tooth, particularly if discovered in an older person, may be left in the jawbone unless it flares up, causing pain and swelling.

Nonimpacted wisdom teeth that do not occlude cannot be used for chewing and are extremely difficult to clean. Consequently, they tend to decay and infect the next molar. Since they frequently contribute to periodontal disease and early loss of the second molars, it is often advisable to have these quite useless teeth removed as part of a good preventive program.

Other teeth can also become impacted. A smaller tooth can be imbedded under the roots of larger teeth, or a tooth can be impacted on its side. Impaction is frequently caused by underdeveloped jaws. Underdevelopment can result from a diet of soft foods that do not require sufficient chewing and grinding before swallowing.

An oddity is the supernumerary, a tooth nobody asked for. It may be any size, any shape and it may erupt at any time, though usually during early childhood. Or, like some wisdom teeth, it may lie unnoticed a lifetime (although it will show up on an x ray). Frequently a supernumerary makes its entrance between the two upper front teeth. The next most common supernumerary is a fourth molar.

Forestalling Problems

None of us have perfect teeth. There is always something awry—a space between the two front teeth, crowding, a crooked incisor, a poor bite or an impacted wisdom tooth.

Consider the space between the two front teeth. If they are primary teeth, the space is welcome. When larger permanent teeth come in, they will need that extra space. If, at age 10 or 12, the teeth are slightly crowded, there's no need to rush to an orthodontist. Human jaws continue to grow until adulthood and they are quite likely to extend in length enough to accommodate all the permanent teeth without crowding.

A crooked tooth usually is the result of overcrowding or heredity, or both. If a child inherits the small jaws of his mother and the large teeth of his father, his teeth may be overcrowded and will, of necessity, overlap one another. Orthodontic work often is considered the remedy.

Improper bites (malocclusions) are conditions in which upper and lower teeth fail to meet as they should, thus contributing to poorly chewed food, increased cavities, periodontal troubles, early loss of teeth and speech defects. Furthermore, a protruding or underslung jaw can bring on emotional upsets among children and, if not corrected, the condition may lead to a life of physical and mental misery. While heredity is often to blame for improperly matched lower and upper jaws, the guilt also falls on thumbsucking carried on beyond an early age and upon poor prenatal and postnatal nutrition. Taking your child to see the dentist early in life can be rewarding, as some malocclusion problems may be forestalled or corrected without lengthy and costly treatments.

Now that you know something about your teeth, we suggest you go to a drugstore and buy an inexpensive mouth mirror with a long handle, similar to the one the dentist uses. The plastic type is less expensive than the metal and just as good for your purposes. Look at your teeth using the mouth mirror and a hand mirror. Inspect each tooth. Use the chart of permanent teeth earlier in this chapter to indicate fillings and mark if there's something about a premolar, for example, that you don't understand. Note the dental work that has been done, how it looks and feels. Really get acquainted with your teeth. They are not just little pieces of bone stuck in the gums. They are living parts of your body, with tissues, nerves and blood vessels, just as alive as your fingers, eyes and heart. Always remember that your mouth is a highly sensitive organ with numerous sensitive nerves.

2 ALLIED SYSTEMS

There's more in your mouth than meets the eye

Many people think only of their teeth when they think of oral care. Teeth are only one important facet in the network: they rely heavily on the supportive structures, without which they'd be totally useless to you, and work with allied mouth systems to enable you to speak, to chew, to swallow, to yawn. In this chapter, we'll explore the interrelationships of mouth organs and discuss them individually.

Chewing and Speaking

We must eat to survive and, to eat a proper diet, we must chew our food so that it can be digested. It involves teeth and gums, jaws, jaw joints and muscles. Then there is the entire supporting system which holds the teeth in place, the lining of the mouth, the little glands which produce saliva and saliva itself.

Infants, like puppies, will bite at and chew almost anything within reach or sight from pure instinct. Unlike puppies, however, little children do not master the art of chewing until they have all their primary teeth. Even then, many a child will need help in eating properly. He must become accustomed to moving his tongue sideways for chewing instead of backward for sucking, to accept harder and larger pieces of food, to learn how long to chew before swallowing and how and when to close his lips.

The mastication process isn't simple: Here's the way it works. A piece of food enters your mouth. Instantly, certain nerves are triggered, signals are flashed to teeth, tongue, cheeks, saliva glands and jaw muscles. The tongue, lips and cheeks start tossing food around between upper and lower teeth. Sprays of saliva moisten and partially digest the food at the same time. (Were it not for saliva, chewing would be impossible. Have you ever tried it when your mouth was dry?) As food is chewed, it breaks down into small, juicy pieces.

When food is sufficiently masticated and lubricated, it lands on your tongue. The tongue shovels it back against the hard palate. While the larynx quickly closes like a trap door, the tongue flips the food down the esophagus. After the food passes, the larynx opens and you can breathe again.

How do the jaws and teeth actually perform their duties? Four muscles start moving with a rotary action and the jaws begin cutting thrusts, as upper and lower teeth gnash away. Biscuspids give a few chomps and then send the food to the molars. When upper and lower molars crunch down on food, the action is similar to the grinding action of a mortar and pestle.

Chewing takes place on one side at a time, although many people like to alternate from side to side. Take a moment to pop something chewy into your mouth. Start chomping, but slowly. Notice how busy the jaws become, how your teeth are constantly in motion, how your tongue is hustling food from one part of your mouth to another. When you have finished chewing, your lower jaw will hang quietly at rest position without upper and lower teeth touching. In fact, that's the way teeth should be most of the time, except for swallowing. Each time you swallow, your teeth contact.

Teeth, tongue, cheeks, lips and jawbones also play essential roles in our ability to speak. How often have you heard someone talk with a whistling sound or a nasal tone? In a normal mouth, this doesn't happen. But if the teeth are not positioned properly or a denture is too thick in the palate, air passage becomes wrongly deflected and this causes funny sounds. These conditions can be eliminated by cosmetic repositioning of the teeth, orthodontic treatment, construction of prosthetic devices and correct dental work. Missing teeth or poorly aligned or spaced teeth can affect the clarity of speech.

Actors, singers and politicians are most aware of the fact that any abnormal condition in their mouths can influence the quality and tone of their voices. Proper speech results when the voice is modified by movements of the pharynx, tongue, lips and cheeks. These movements are controlled by special centers in the brain. Speech would be impossible without the moistening and lubricating effects of saliva.

Periodontal Tissues

GINGIVA

In the first chapter, we described how the tooth is rooted in periodontal tissues and how, without those tissues, the tooth would have neither anchor nor support. Let's discuss periodontal tissues, or periodontium, a little further. *Periodontium* consists of four separate tissues: the gingiva, the alveolar process, the periodontal ligament, and the cementum. Cementum is discussed under tooth structure in Chapter 1.

As the gums go, so go the teeth. To protect and save them, one must brush teeth and gums and floss daily. Also, inspect them regularly and get treatment for them immediately at the first sign of change. To better understand your gums, it is important to invest in a mouth mirror and thereby get a closer look. There is one on the market with a small attached flashlight. To prevent your mirror from fogging up when your breath hits it, first rinse the mirror in warm water.

What do you know about gums and their functions? Properly

called gingiva, gums are the tissues that surround the necks of teeth and parts of jaws, and are classified as periodontal tissue. This gingiva tightly hugs the teeth and helps to hold them in place. Between each tooth there is a small triangular section of firm gum tissue.

When examining your gums with a dental mirror, do not be alarmed if you notice a few blood vessels or the bridge of a bone under the gum. Blood vessels, especially in fair-skinned people, often are visible and that bone is merely the root of your tooth. Perfectly normal. While you are exploring, be sure to look at the backs of your teeth and gums—the lingual surfaces. These are the surfaces people often neglect, thinking no one will see them anyway.

Gingiva aids greatly in holding your teeth in place. The tight, knifelike edge around each tooth prevents food or other foreign matter from dropping between tooth and gum. Gums can protect your teeth from injury and bacteria. And the more rough work you give your gums, such as crunching down on celery sticks, the better your gums will like it.

Healthy gingiva is usually described as light pink or coral. Variations in gingival color seem to be correlated to the complexion and the degree of skin pigmentation of the individual.

Almost everyone, at some time in life, has discovered a spot of pink on his or her toothbrush or when rinsing the mouth. This slight bleeding from the gingiva may last only a day or two. Or it may continue and increase. In any instance, bleeding gums should never be neglected, for this is a sign that something is wrong and the sooner the problem is corrected the better off you will be.

Bleeding is caused by a gum inflammation which in turn may be due to any number of things: deposits of plaque or tartar or food debris, or an injurious blow to the gingiva. The body tries to defend itself from irritation by mobilizing an army of red and white blood cells to fight off the bacteria in plaque and tartar. As the blood cells rush into the site of irritation, inflammation flares up and the tiny capillaries become overextended, like a balloon ready to burst. The slightest touch of a toothbrush or vigorous rinsing can cause these capillaries to break open. And that's how your gums begin to bleed. Your next step, of course, is to make an appointment with your dentist and find out what is wrong.

Failure to give at least 15 minutes a day to cleaning teeth and gums in at least two sessions can undoubtedly bring on a gum problem. Fortunately, early gum problems usually can be healed within 4 or 5 weeks, but only if a meticulous home dental care schedule is followed.

There are many stages of gum disease and, all too often, individuals will let their gums progressively deteriorate from one stage to the next before seeking help. The longer one procrastinates, the worse the gums will be and the higher the dental bills.

With conscientious care, you should have very little trouble with gums. However, there is a condition called *gingival recession.* This is a falling away of relatively healthy gums from the necks of the teeth. It may be caused by an incorrect bite or excessive or improper brushing. Gingival recession can happen to anyone at any age. A detailed discussion of diseases of the gingiva and their treatment is provided in Chapter 6.

ALVEOLAR PROCESS

Each tooth lies in its own socket. The alveolar process is the bone that forms and supports the sockets of the teeth. The fascinating thing about the alveolar bone is that it is constantly being dissolved and reformed as a result of the pressure and tension to which it is subjected. For example, when a tooth gets moved into a new position, as in orthodontic correction, bone is resorbed at the wall of the socket where pressure is being exerted and is formed on the opposite wall.

Trouble comes to the alveolar process when upper and lower teeth are poorly aligned. Chewing is uneven, causing stress to fall heavily on certain teeth and passing up others. The little bones in the sockets cannot cope with this kind of erratic treatment and, in time, bones are absorbed and teeth get loose and fall out.

PERIODONTAL LIGAMENT

Thin, rugged connective tissue fibers form the periodontal ligament. This ligament attaches the roots of your teeth to their sockets, supports the teeth, attaches the gums to teeth and acts as a shock absorber during mastication. It's a great aid in telling which tooth hurts, especially if the tooth contacts something hot or cold.

Periodontal ligament varies from one individual to another and the thickness seems to increase with usage and decrease with less usage.

Tongue and Lips

The tongue is a muscular organ; its mucous membrane contains three different kinds of taste buds, numbering some 3,000 in all. A person tastes sweets on the top of the tongue, bitter on the back, sour and salt usually on the sides. The tongue also has its own nerve, through which it transfers touch, pain and temperature; it is essential for chewing, swallowing and speaking. The tongue is a very strong organ for its size. You've heard that old expression, "with tongue in cheek." Just press your tongue against your cheek and see if you can still smile!

Without muscles in the lips, no one would ever be able to keep food inside his mouth. Luckily, we possess an assortment of facial muscles. Some extend from the cheek wall into the lip, others connect lips and cheeks to the jaws. And there are muscles in the floor of the mouth, all necessary for chewing and speaking.

Nervous and Circulatory Systems

Like the rest of your body, your mouth contains an intricate network of nerves supplying teeth, lower jaw, the skin of your chin and lower lip. Your mouth is also supplied with a splendid circulatory system. Several arteries are constantly pulsating around in your head and at least four of them send blood directly to palate, tongue, chin, lips, muscles of mastication and into the deep areas of the upper jaw. That's how gums get their blood supply and why they sometimes may bleed, which they normally should not do.

Mucous Membranes

Nature thoughtfully lined our mouths with a material similar to the mucous membrane linings in other body cavities. Called *mucosa,* this is the lining visible inside lips and cheeks and under the tongue. It is a soft, pinkish tissue, easily injured when you accidentally bite the inside of your cheek. But the mucosa repairs itself quickly. The oral mucosa has many blood and lymph vessels; mucous-producing glands are lodged deep inside.

Salivary Glands

Two salivary glands lie under the tongue and they have ducts which squirt out saliva. There are larger glands located just under the skin in front of and under each ear. Still other small ducts are on the floor of your mouth and all of them work around the clock to keep your mouth moistened.

Did you ever wonder why saliva tends to flood your mouth whenever you sit back in a dental chair? Any physical stimulus in your mouth—whether a stick of chewing gum or a dentist's finger—immediately activates the salivary glands. We know that the flow of saliva is also increased when we're hungry, when we peer into a bakery window, when we smell something delicious cooking. Even the thought of food can become a mouth-watering experience.

Saliva is a secretion which is mostly water with a small amount of mucous and other substances. As an aid to mastication, saliva is indispensable because, without some form of lubrication for the food, chewing and swallowing would be impossible. Also, saliva carries an enzyme which begins digesting carbohydrates even before they are swallowed. Other substances in saliva act in antibacterial and buffering ways to prevent the mouth from becoming too acid or too alkaline. The composition of saliva not only varies from one individual to the next, it may even vary from one minute to the next. It is so accomodating that, should you be eating a potato and suddenly switch to a piece of steak, saliva will automatically thicken to make the steak easier to chew.

It is known that tooth decay and periodontal disease can increase if there should be a deficiency in the amount of saliva produced; the quantity may be influenced by an individual's health. In a healthy body, saliva is one of nature's remarkable ways of cleaning teeth and gums and also holding the line against destruction by certain harmful bacteria. Your teeth are being bathed constantly in a fresh supply of saliva, which is not only good for your mouth and your digestion, but certainly makes it easier for you to speak and smile. Will your saliva ever run dry? It's unlikely. The average person produces about three pints daily.

3 NUTRITION AND HYGIENE
Saving your own teeth

Your dentist alone cannot keep your teeth healthy and your mouth in good shape. He cannot correct in two hours the damage done by months or years of neglect on your part. Good nutrition and a daily hygienic routine are absolute musts—a major part of the battle in keeping your teeth sound for a lifetime. Even if you have badly neglected oral hygiene through the years, it is never too late to institute a routine of care that can substantially alleviate any problems you have. Three months of diligent home care can put an average individual's mouth into a healthy state. Three months of neglect can put it back into a sorry state. The benefits of good hygienic and nutritional patterns will manifest themselves in other ways, as well. Just as poor oral health affects the rest of your body adversely, the reverse is also true: good oral health is part and parcel of a vigorous physical condition.

This study illustrates the importance of your role in saving your own teeth. Some 20 years ago, a group of twelve dentists in New Jersey began an experimental program of preventive dentistry. They started out with new ground rules. Instead of short, insufficient sessions with children after school, every child arrived in the early morning, fresh and good natured, when the dentist could spend more time. Many hours were given to restoring young patients' mouths to healthy states. With medication, anesthetics and even hypnotism, pain was almost nil. Root canal therapy and other treatments saved tooth after tooth. More hours were given to teaching and demonstrating home care. A major project, but would it work?

Not immediately. Only half the battle was won. The dentists had done their part. Now it was up to the parents and the children. At the very beginning, dentists explained that they were providing knowledge, skill, labor and time. Parents were paying the bills. Would it be worth all the dentists' efforts and all the parents' investments if the childrens' mouths lapsed back to their former neglected conditions? And if the entire procedure had to be repeated? "No!" the dentists flatly declared. If the program was to work, it had to have each child's unconditional cooperation or the dentists would no longer treat the patient.

What the dentists wanted was a three-way program. First: a dentist would teach each child how to brush correctly and how to eat the right kind of food. Second: the parents would keep a close check on the child. If the child was too young, a parent coached by the dentist would care for the child's mouth. Third: if fluoride was not already in the drinking water, fluoride was to be applied to the teeth. If cavities continued, a special decay-control diet planned by the School of Dentistry at the University of Michigan was suggested.

It worked! Checkups showed a marked reduction in cavities. Gradually, young patients required less dental work, with most of their visits only to the hygienist. The biggest surprise came when adults began asking for the same program. Delighted, the dentists instructed them in oral hygienic routine and insisted on thorough examination, tooth repairs and replacements if needed, regular scaling and cleaning. The adults who followed the program were amazed. Some had no new cavities at all, some had only one or two small ones. The few who might have lost teeth discovered that their teeth had been saved.

There is no reason why everyone should not have all their

teeth in excellent condition throughout a lifetime. They are your teeth and surely you want to keep them.

Sound Nutrition for Sound Teeth

A BASIC PLAN

The food we eat is extremely important. People can be healthy on many diets, but most dentists recommend that, to maintain cavity-free teeth, a balanced, nutritious diet should be made up from the four basic categories: *dairy products; fruits and vegetables; meat, poultry* and *fish; grains.*

For a healthy body and healthy teeth, you may want to plan a diet for yourself. Select from each of the four food groups, allowing two or more servings of dairy products; one or two fruits; at least one leafy vegetable and one non-leafy vegetable; two or more servings from the meat, poultry and fish group; four or more servings of grain products.

According to the Department of Agriculture, half the people in American households are not eating well. The major deficits were found to be a lack of vitamins A and C and calcium (all needed for healthy teeth and gums).

What can be done about it?

We can start by reeducating ourselves. Don't be lured by advertising into buying products you know little about. Cut out "junk foods," such as potato chips and cola drinks, processed foods, frozen dinners, candies, ice cream. Most lack sufficient nutrients and many contain controversial preservatives and additives. Particularly be aware of sugar-loaded breakfast cereals, which entice children via TV commercials. If your child demands these attractive but dentally harmful products, explain why they are not allowed and be firm in your refusal to purchase them. Buy unsugared cereals instead—they're cheaper in more ways than one.

A RADICAL PLAN FOR RADICAL IMPROVEMENT

Too many of us are "carboholics," constantly eating white bread, doughnuts, macaroni, dumplings, hotcakes (with lots of syrup), chocolate bars, sugar in coffee, a second piece of that good old American apple pie. Most carboholics, adults and children, have a number of fillings, but there is a way to get rid of that harmful craving. It's the University of Michigan's low-carbohydrate diet which should be supervised by a hygienist. The plan lasts six weeks and it is broken into three phases of two weeks each. Briefly, it goes like this:

Phase one (first and second weeks): All refined sugars and starches are forbidden. No bread, potatoes, cakes, pies, candy, cookies or soft drinks. You may eat all the meat, poultry, fruits, vegetables, and milk or milk products you want.

Phase two (third and fourth weeks): A few carbohydrates, such as potatoes and bread, are allowed. All the meats, fish, poultry, fruits, vegetables and milk are still available.

Phase three (fifth and sixth weeks): Sugar in whatever form desired may be eaten each day at one meal and *one meal only.*

Here's a great tip: if you must have sugar in your daily diet, whether the sugar is in a beverage, dessert or candy, phase three shows you the smartest way to consume it. Experiments have proved that *the amount of sugar eaten is not as important as the frequency.* If you eat the same amount of sugar in any form ten times a day, that sugar will attack your teeth ten times instead of once. So go ahead and splurge. Once. Then brush your teeth and floss thoroughly.

Even better is the habit of eating hard, tough "detergent" foods, such as tough meat, hard bread, raw vegetables and raw fruits which make you chew and tear at your food. It may sound barbaric, but that's the way our ancestors ate and that's the way dentists would like us to continue to eat in order to stimulate circulation in gums and to tone up gum tissues, just as one might tone up the muscles in their arms and legs. A nice, crisp apple a day may help to keep also the dentist away.

The Vitamin Connection

Some dentists, physicians and dieticians say we get all the vitamins required if we eat well-balanced diets. We will then have the necessary amounts of vitamins A, B, C and D, which help in building good teeth and gums, and we will get into trouble only when we fail to drink orange juice or milk. But lately, dentists and physicians researching and experimenting in preventive dentistry have come up with some surprises.

Emanuel Cheraskin, M.D., D.D.S., professor at the University of Alabama's School of Dentistry, believes nutrition is important in building up resistance to plaque diseases and he has proved that resistance is influenced by a patient's vitamin intake. To test the effect of vitamin C supplements on the health of gum tissues, a group of volunteers was assembled and their gums carefully examined. Half of the group received vitamin C daily. The other half received placebo pills. Each subject received a thorough scaling on one side of the mouth. That resulted in four different groups: (1) Scaling with vitamin C; (2) No scaling with vitamin C; (3) Scaling with placebos; (4) No scaling with placebos. Three weeks later, all mouths were reexamined. The gum conditions had improved significantly in three out of four groups. The mouths of the group that had nothing were in the worst shape. Those who had either scaling or vitamin C were a little better. The fourth group, which had received both scaling and vitamin C, showed the greatest improvement in gingival health.

In other experiments, Dr. Cheraskin observed that injuries to the gums healed twice as fast with the intake of vitamin C and even faster if other vitamins were added.

Many highly regarded dentists agree with Dr. Cheraskin that, together with home care, increased vitamin C helps prevention of plaque and tartar deposits. Some progressive dentists are prescribing individualized diets with a proper balance of vitamins for their patients. The results have been amazing. Dentists have realized a significant reduction of cavities among their patients and, looking into the future, they anticipate the prevention of 99 percent of cavities.

If you should need heavy doses of vitamin C, swallow the tablets instead of sucking them. Continuous contact with the ascorbic acid in vitamin C tablets can cause erosion to tooth enamel. Also, frequent intake of orange juice will keep your teeth bathed in acid and predispose them to decay (enjoy your juice through a straw).

Fluoridation

Fluoridation is one more important aid to keeping your teeth. Children drinking naturally or artificially fluoridated water have had 50 to 60 percent fewer instances of dental decay than those not drinking fluoridated water. If your community does not provide fluoridated water, you might consider taking the children to a dentist or hygienist well trained in applying topical fluoride. The fluoride solution is applied to the teeth with a swab or a specially designed tray that fits in the mouth, filled with fluoride preparations, and is finished in a few minutes. Usually four such treatments are given at one-week intervals at the ages of 3, 7, 11 and 13. A fluoride solution is also applied to teeth at the end of each cleaning session in the dentist's office.

Fluoride retards tooth decay primarily because it is incorporated into the tooth enamel before permanent teeth erupt. The enamel hardens and is resistant to acid and decay. In adults, fluoride hardens the tooth surface, making it more resistant to bacteria. There have been instances where fluoridated water proved itself capable of warding off cavities well into middle age and stopped then only because of encroaching periodontal diseases.

Highly concentrated fluoride in water can be harmful and can cause teeth to become mottled. One should not attempt to use a self-administered fluoride, either in tablet or liquid form, except with the advice and supervision of a dentist and hygienist.

The American Dental Association will not allow a toothpaste with fluoride to carry its seal of approval until the ADA has thoroughly checked and tested the manufacturer's formula and the dentifrice proves to have therapeutic value.

Fluoride on top of fluoride: isn't it a bit too much? Scientific studies show that individuals who live in areas with fluoridated water *and* use fluoridated toothpaste have less dental disease than individuals in the same areas not using fluoridated toothpaste. Fluoride in toothpaste is different than fluoride in water. It affects the teeth as an additive, i.e., it works externally, rather than internally.

Fluoride toothpastes do help, but the results can be many times better with careful and frequent brushing. ADA-approved fluoridated toothpastes state right on the tube: ". . . can be of significant value when used in a conscientiously applied program of oral hygiene and regular professional care."

Daily Hygienic Routines

We advocate that you brush your teeth three times a day, following each meal, and floss thoroughly at least once a day. However, your own dentist may feel that this is too rigid a program and place all his emphasis on a *thorough* brushing once a day. It takes 24 hours for bacteria to reorganize into plaque and for the plaque to attach itself to a tooth after it has been scraped off. Therefore, many dental authorities believe that one significant cleaning session a day is adequate. You and your dentist should arrive at the best possible plan for you: seek his advice and then *follow it.* The daily hygienic routine is your best chance to save yourself money, pain and time.

Here is a list of the items adults should have to keep teeth clean and gums healthy.

Toothbrushes
Toothpaste with fluoride
Dental floss or dental tape
  (buy a large size—you'll need it)
Disclosing tablets or solution
Dental mirror (or a good magnifying hand mirror)
Oral irrigating device
Electric toothbrush (optional)
Salt

For children, supply the same items except the brushes should be smaller. And omit the oral irrigating device if the children are quite young.

Toothbrushing

MANUAL AND ELECTRIC TOOTHBRUSHES

It is more accurate and descriptive to call a toothbrush a *tooth-gum brush* because it is used to brush and massage gum tissues as well as teeth. Purchase three or four so you can rotate, allowing each brush to dry for 24 hours before being used again. The brushes will last longer. A collapsible travel brush you can carry in pocket or purse if you're having lunch or dinner out is a good idea. Never use old, worn brushes. Replace brushes often, as soon as old ones show signs of wear. Brushes need to be replaced about four times a year, more often for children, who tend to chew on the bristles.

Buy brushes with straight handles, flat brushing surfaces, and soft or medium rounded and polished bristles for minimal gingival trauma. Advocated brushing techniques today utilize a soft-bristle brush. Too stiff a brush can lacerate delicate gingival tissues.

Studies of bristle abrasiveness on tooth structures have shown that there is little or no abrasive effect on enamel and dentin, whether the brush is made of natural or synthetic bristles. Abrasion of tooth structure is independent of the stiffness or the composition of the bristle, but depends almost entirely on the abrasive properties of the paste or powder used on the toothbrush. For example, a medium abrasive toothpowder will increase the abrasive action of any toothbrush by several hundred percent.

Natural bristles were popular in the past. When the war interfered with their sources of supply, nylon bristles were developed. With the passing of time, nylon bristles have been greatly improved and are precisely manufactured. Nylon bristles last longer, will not easily become soggy or soft. They will not split or fray and are more easily cleaned.

Electric toothbrushes should not be overlooked, as they have become quite popular in the last two decades. But are they good for your teeth? Yes and no. The type that brushes vertically—up and down—is considered acceptable. Its brush is small enough to reach into difficult-to-reach areas and it also removes stains and plaque better than the hand brush. On the negative side, because any powered toothbrush tends to wear tooth structures, it is recommended that you use this brush only once a day.

Also on the market are electric toothbrushes that move horizontally—back and forth—but they are not in line with the currently suggested method of brushing, so they are not considered desirable.

An electric toothbrush can be extremely helpful to handicapped persons and children. Anyone having difficulty using their arms or hands will find the powered model a boon. Children will at first become intrigued with the mechanism of the toothbrush and, when the novelty wears off, they will be more apt to do a good cleansing job in less time than brushing manually. The younger the child, the shorter the attention span; that's why a speedy electric toothbrush is welcome.

Remember that children's brushes are softer, children struggle more trying to properly manipulate the brush and, consequently, their toothbrushes wear out faster than do those of adults.

TOOTHPASTES

Buy whichever fluoride paste tastes best and leaves your mouth feeling freshest. Some fluoridated toothpastes, including Crest, Colgate and MacLeans, have been given the seal of acceptance from the American Dental Association (see Fluoridation, earlier in this chapter). Homemade dentrifrices, such as salt-and-baking-soda mixtures, are generally too abrasive. They can wear down tooth enamel and cause excessive erosion; they are not considered desirable.

BRUSHING TECHNIQUES

There are two main techniques advised for brushing the primary teeth and mixed dentition, and at least seven major brushing techniques for adult teeth.

Studies have shown that no one method is clearly superior to others; rather, the thoroughness of plaque and debris removal is achieved by the careful and correct application of an acceptable technique. Your dentist or periodontist will likely recommend a brushing method based on an evaluation of your individual needs.

For most of us, it is best to learn a method that is not excessively difficult or complicated, and that will do an adequate job of stimulating the gingival tissues as well as cleansing plaque and debris from the teeth. First learn the basic brushing method most prescribed to remove plaque without using toothpaste on the brush. Remember, it is the complete removal of plaque without damaging the gums and teeth that is important.

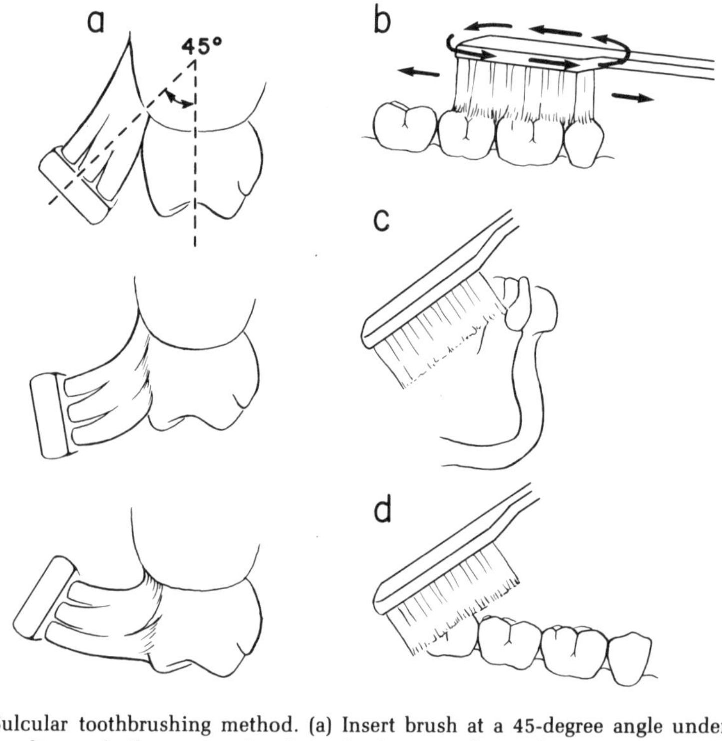

Sulcular toothbrushing method. (a) Insert brush at a 45-degree angle under gumline and vibrate, then brush in the direction the tooth grows. Clean only two or three teeth at a time. (b) Chewing surfaces are brushed with a vibrating, circular motion combined with short back-and-forth strokes. (c) To brush the lingual surfaces of the front teeth, hold brush at a 45-degree angle. Insert the last three or four rows of bristles under the gumline and vibrate and move the brush in a heel-to-toe direction. (d) To clean the back of the last molar, press brush over the chewing surface and down against the gum, then vibrate.

Hold your brush firmly at a 45-degree angle and place the brush parallel with the surface of the teeth. Start with your front teeth. They're easiest to watch. The bristle ends should be pointed just over the gumline, with the sides of the bristles touching the gingival tissues. Now rotate the brush slowly and gently with short strokes, moving the bristles toward the occlusal, or chewing, surface. Use enough pressure to feel the bristles scrubbing your gums.

Try brushing this way on all outer surfaces of your teeth and then move to the inside surfaces, using the same vibrating, rotating, up-and-down action.

For the lingual, or back, surfaces of the front teeth, which are more difficult to reach, you must hold your brush vertically at the same 45-degree angle, but with the front part of the brush touching the gums. Brush the inside front of the teeth, both uppers and lowers, by moving the brush in a heel-to-toe direction.

The chewing surfaces of your teeth also should be brushed with the scrubbing action, moving the brush horizontally from back to front. Press the bristles down firmly and move the brush back and forth with short strokes. If you find it tight getting to the back molars, angle the brush on the molars and close your jaws slightly. You'll find you have more room. A newly designed brush with a slight angle came on the market recently and seems to reach the back molars quite easily.

If periodontitis is present, an extra brushing procedure is needed to remove plaque accumulations in the gingival sulcus and interproximal spaces. With the bristle ends pointed just above the gumline, the brush handle is vibrated gently and rapidly, forcing the bristles into the interproximal spaces. This procedure will clean the interproximal spaces, as well as massaging gingival tissues.

Never brush back and forth horizontally on any tooth surfaces except the biting surfaces. Brushing back and forth on other surfaces can injure your gums and wear away tooth enamel, causing abrasion and erosion at the necks of your teeth. Remember to brush your teeth the way they grow, from neck to chewing surface.

A good idea is to map out a pattern of brushing before you begin. Divide your upper and lower dental arches into five sections—two sections on each side and one in the middle. Start brushing on the outside of your upper left molars, giving them at least ten strokes. Go on to the next section and repeat the brushing. Then the center. Follow around to the right side, finishing at the right molars. Always ten strokes for each section.

Repeat with the outside of your lower arch. Following the same pattern, brush the inside sections of your upper arch and then the lower arch. Polish off by scrubbing the biting surfaces. Go back to the uppers and repeat the ten-stroke procedure. Then go to the lowers and repeat. Then the third time around. Five or six minutes should give you an adequate cleaning job. An egg timer can be an excellent inexpensive reminder of how long you have brushed. Add toothpaste and start brushing, working your way around your mouth slowly, carefully and correctly. Every once in a while, rinse with warm water. And don't forget to brush the top of your tongue, because there are many crevices on the tongue which retain countless bacteria and debris. If you are not sure how to brush your teeth correctly, your dentist, dental assistant or hygienist will gladly demonstrate.

Flossing

DENTAL FLOSSES AND TAPES

There are many types of floss and tape on the market, including unwaxed, waxed and partially waxed. Many dentists prefer dental tape, which is wider and seems to be more effective in cleaning between the teeth. If contact between teeth is very tight, the floss will slip through easier.

Unwaxed floss is probably the most effective in removing plaque. It produces a squeaky sound when the tooth surface is clean. It does not leave wax residue on the tooth. However, some people find the unwaxed type difficult to use, as it tends to shred or break when they pass it through tight contacts. Waxed floss seems easier to handle and tends to resist shredding. It would be best to purchase small rolls of the various types to try out; learn which of these works best for you before you purchase the more costly larger sizes.

There are various instruments on the market, such as interproximal brushes, floss threaders and stimulators, for cleaning

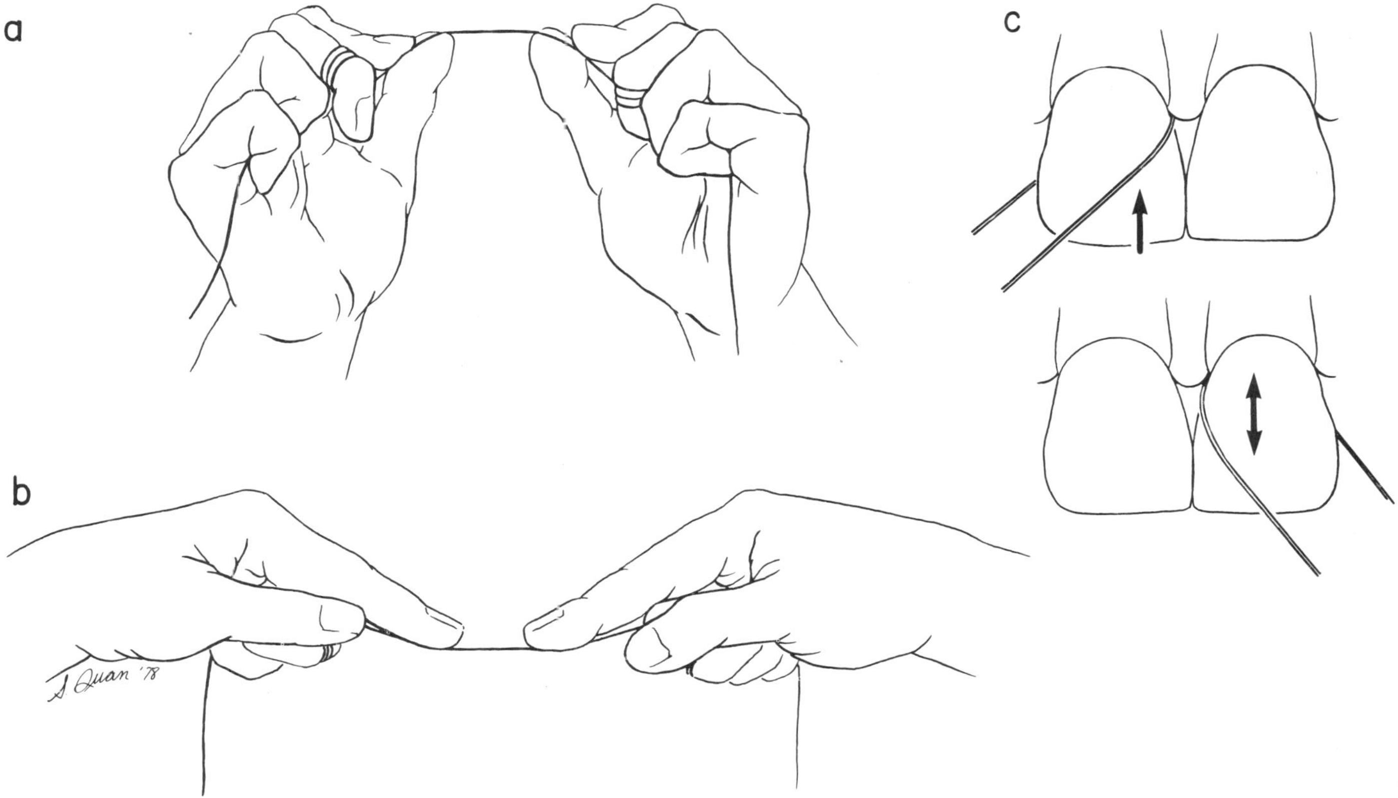

Flossing. (a) Wrapping the floss around the middle fingers; for upper teeth, use thumb and index fingers to hold the floss. (b) For lower teeth, use index fingers to hold floss. (c) Insert floss between teeth, using a gentle sawing motion. Wrap the floss around the tooth. Scrape up and down the side of one tooth until a squeaking sound is heard. Repeat on the side of the other tooth.

between a fixed bridge and the gums, but get your dentist's approval before using them. Also let him show you how to use these aids; otherwise, you might damage or loosen expensive bridgework.

FLOSSING TECHNIQUES

After adequate brushing, it's flossing time. Undoubtedly, the major lack in most oral hygiene programs is the inadequate use of dental floss. Flossing is the best way known to remove plaque and food particles from between your teeth and around the gumline. These are the difficult, hidden areas that your toothbrush cannot reach. But they should be reached at least every 24 hours. If you have never used dental floss, you may find the going a little tricky. But it's worth learning. Here is the easiest and best technique.

Pull out about 18 inches of dental floss or dental tape from the dispenser and wind one end around your right middle finger and the other end around your left middle finger. Wrap most of the floss on one finger, because when you start flossing, the opposite finger will act as a take-up reel as the floss becomes soiled. Leave only a short length between middle fingers and another short length of floss between both thumbs, which will act as guides.

Watch yourself in a mirror. Curl your upper lip and work just on the upper front teeth. Hold the floss taut, thumbs and index fingers guiding as you apply a gentle sawing motion to insert the floss between two teeth. Never push down hard or snap the floss into the gums. Carefully wiggle the floss past the contact area. When the floss reaches your gumline, wrap the floss around one tooth and tenderly slide it down under the gumline. Still holding the floss tightly, scrape up and down against the tooth, working toward the contact point. Wrap the floss around the other tooth and repeat the procedure. When the sides of both teeth are cleaned, let out some clean floss and reel up the slack on the other finger. Now seesaw the clean floss upward, past the contact point and out. Repeat the procedure with all other upper teeth. When you have finished, rinse vigorously with warm water to wash out loose plaque and debris.

When you start on the lower teeth, turn your hands downward and guide the floss with the index fingers only. Proceed to clean the lower teeth in the same fashion. The technique may be a little awkward at first, but you catch on with practice.

The ADA suggests you divide your mouth into four sections. Floss half of your upper teeth, then the other half, and repeat with the lower quadrants. Establishing a regular flossing pattern prevents missing any part of your mouth. Don't forget to floss around the back surface of your posterior teeth, which do not have any teeth behind them. This area is often overlooked. It is also important to set a certain time for daily flossing so that you won't forget. Bedtime is the most popular hour, but many dentists would like to see you brush and floss after each meal.

Flossing is a skill that takes time to develop. Your dentist will certainly show you how to floss and help you develop the correct technique. Some people have teeth that are far apart and, if yours are like that, go in cautiously with the dental floss to avoid injuring gum tissue. If some of your teeth are so crowded that it is impossible to wiggle floss between them, then—according to one school of dentistry—food can't get there either, so forget it. Other dentists may show you how to thread floss between two crowded teeth. Some dentists prefer flossing before brushing. After you have finished flossing, place a small amount of water in your mouth and move that water forcefully around and between your teeth to dislodge any food particles which might still remain. An oral irrigating unit, if you own one, will do the same job more effectively.

Lastly, if your gums become slightly sore and bleed a little the first days you use floss, don't panic. It's all part of cleaning up plaque and debris. Of course, if soreness and bleeding continue more than a week, something else is wrong. Go to your dentist.

Some dentists may recommend the use of interdental stimulators for cleaning between teeth and for stimulation or circulation of the gingival tissue. Interdental stimulators are made of splinterless wooden sticks, triangular in cross section and pointed at the working end, which fit well into the space between the teeth.

Cleaning Aids: Pro and Con

Incorrectly used for long periods, toothpicks can mechanically wear tooth structure and injure the gums, resulting in periodontal disease. A toothpick may also break, leaving its tip embedded between the teeth, causing severe inflammation. Resorption of alveolar bone has been observed in people who keep a toothpick wedged between their teeth constantly. If you need to remove something between your teeth, use floss!

There are many useful preventive products and cleaning aids available: tiny brushes to go between the teeth or between exposed roots; dental swabs and applicators, to be moistened with disclosing solutions and applied to teeth and gingival margins and for cleaning hard-to-reach areas.

Have rubber tips on the ends of toothbrushes ever puzzled you? Supposedly, they are made to massage your gums and clean between your teeth. They do loosen plaque more or less, but are not as useful as generally thought.

ORAL IRRIGATING DEVICES

An oral irrigating device is among the dental items you should have on hand. These devices come in two types. One is the electric type that sends out pulsating jets of water to cleanse around the gums and between teeth where the toothbrush and even floss sometimes cannot reach. The other type is not electric and attaches to a faucet. Most dentists believe every home should have the device and they favor the electric model; water pressure and temperature can be easily regulated.

The dental irrigator is not recommended for small children, but for children over 12 years with orthodontic bands, the device is a godsend. The stream of water directed at the bands is invaluable in flushing out food particles. For adults with gum problems, the water not only cleans between the teeth, under fixed bridges and around gums, but will also massage gums and stimulate circulation.

Instructions for an oral irrigating device will accompany the machine, but it would be wise to check with your dentist before use, as everyone has different needs. Basically, you fill the machine's container with lukewarm water, aim the tip of a small hose at your gumline, adjust to the pressure desired, turn on the device and let the jets of water travel along the gumline on the outside and inside surfaces. You may be surprised at the amount of debris that rushes out.

An important caution is not to turn the pressure to maximum strength, for it may loosen some bridgework or cause some marginal fillings to fall out. An advantage of the electric irrigating device is that it carries several plastic tips, which means a family can use the same machine but each person will have his own personal tip.

The irrigating device should be used once a day at minimum, particularly if you have bridgework, orthondontic bands or gum problems. Four or five times a week is adequate if your mouth is in great condition. But remember, the irrigating device does *not* take the place of the toothbrush or the dental floss. It does not remove plaque and can only flush out debris after it has been loosened by a brush or floss.

DISCLOSING TABLETS

After you have brushed, flossed and flushed your teeth carefully, your teeth should be in top form, free of plaque. But there is a way to be sure. That's where disclosing tablets, disclosing solution or Plak-Lite come in. They are the detectives who discover the presence of your worst enemy—plaque.

Most popular is the disclosing tablet and the procedure is simple. After you have thoroughly cleaned your teeth, put one of the little red tablets in your mouth, chew it and swish it around for about sixty seconds. Empty your mouth. In case you swallow some of the tablet, don't worry. It is harmless.

Under a good light and with your dental mirror, start the inspection. Your whole mouth, tongue included, will be bright pink, but that's all right. What you must look for is a patch or streak of deep red: the enemy! The disclosing tablet can reveal plaque even on a capped tooth. So it's back to the toothbrush and the dental floss but, at least, you know the areas to attack and you will get them all.

As a beginner, use the disclosing tablet every time you brush and floss. After you have the knack, a spot check once a week should be sufficient. Incidentally, it is quite normal for your tongue and gums to remain colored for a brief period, but the color will wash away.

Disclosing solution is used in the same manner. Probably the easiest to handle, certainly the easiest for children, is the Plak-Lite. After cleansing, you apply three or four drops of disclosing solution under the tongue, work it around the mouth and rinse. Look at your teeth under the Plak-Lite and any remaining plaque will be noticeably yellow.

Mouthwashes

SALT RINSES

Why did we put salt on our "must have" list? Simply because salt makes the best mouthwash available anywhere at any cost—and it's less than a penny a week. Rinsing your mouth several times a day will help sore or inflamed gums. Half a teaspoon of salt in a glass of warm water is all you need. Rinse thoroughly, swishing the salt water between teeth, over them and around them. Then empty your mouth. You'll find the warm salt water soothing. Repeat whenever you feel like it and your gums will thank you. Salt has been a cure-all for centuries.

PEROXIDE MOUTHWASH

Another inexpensive and excellent homemade mouthwash can easily be prepared with 3 percent hydrogen peroxide. The peroxide should be mixed with an equal amount of water: one ounce of hydrogen peroxide plus one ounce of warm water. You can use a measuring cup or an accurate jigger. The therapeutic value of this mouthwash comes from oxygen which, in its bubbly liquid form, dives into every crevice in your mouth, brings oxygen to the cells and kills some of the bacteria. If you're having gum trouble, rinse your mouth two or three times a day, but don't overuse. Do not swallow the mixture. It won't kill you, but it won't make you feel very good.

These two homemade mouthwashes will work better than most present commercial brands and certainly will save you money.

COMMERCIAL PRODUCTS

Commercial mouthwashes can freshen your mouth and your breath for a while, but they will not do much to help your teeth and gums. When manufacturers of commercial mouthwashes ask you to use their products to eliminate bad breath, they are really suggesting that you try to mask unpleasant breath often caused by decayed teeth, diseased gums or some other physical disorder. Moreover, any mouthwash product—at this date—that claims it can remove plaque, prevent decay or gum disease, or can relieve dental pain is a fraud.

Sometimes a mouthwash used excessively can cause more harm than good. There was a young man who had bad breath and his girlfriend told him so. She said, "You'd better get to a dentist, because I think you have cavities."

The young man made a long-overdue appointment with his dentist, but even before arriving at the dentist's office, he bought a bottle of mouthwash and started using it. Just as the patient's girlfriend had predicted, the dentist found three large decayed areas, which he cleaned and filled. Next, the hygienist gave the young man a careful cleaning and scaling and, because his gums were inflamed, he was advised to start immediately on a home care program, carefully described. He was told to return every three months.

Obediently, the young man went to work on home care and regularly kept his appointments with the hygienist. On each visit, both hygienist and dentist shook their heads. If the young man had faithfully carried out his home care program and if the hygienist had thoroughly done her job, why was there a burned appearance in the lining of his mouth? What had gone wrong?

The answer was simple. Because the young man was so afraid of getting bad breath again, he had been using a commercial mouthwash six or seven times a day. What he didn't know was that the mouthwash contained antibacterial ingredients which often kill good bacteria and leave the bad ones to thrive. If mouthwash is applied too many times a day, it can also burn the lining of the mouth.

We sincerely trust that you are motivated to embark at once on your own dental health care program. We believe you do *not* want a sick mouth. Remember three points: proper nutrition, fluoride therapy, plaque control. Plaque removal is your responsibility. If you are a parent, you have a dual responsibility—to yourself and to your child (or children). Certainly there would be no harm in enlisting the rest of your family and friends in the program.

4 PREVENTIVE DENTISTRY
Your dentist and the routine checkup

You have the right to expect high-quality professional work, and that's exactly what you will get if you are knowledgeable about your teeth, prepared to make an intelligent decision on the various treatment plans proposed by your dentist or a specialist to whom he might refer you, and always insist on getting a thorough, logical explanation for any problem that is troubling you. This chapter will tell you how to find a good dentist, how to work with him to get the best results for you, how to evaluate the quality of care you are getting, and what you should expect during a routine checkup.

Getting the Best Professional Care

A good dentist is often more difficult to find than a good physician. Why? Because most physicians are affiliated with hospitals, where they are constantly under the scrutiny of peers. They have greater opportunities to discuss cases and share knowledge with more experienced colleagues. If a physician's work is poor, word gets around. If his work and skill is admired by colleagues, the physician builds up a fine reputation and practice.

We refer to the dentist as "he" only because the majority of dentists in the United States are men. There are women dentists, about 13 percent. More and more are coming into the field, although they are greatly outnumbered by women dentists in Europe, Asia and the USSR. The reverse is happening with dental assistants and hygienists, who have traditionally been women. Now men are taking up the professions.

Even with the growing trend to group practice, where several dentists work in one large office or in a dental clinic setup, most dentists still work alone. A dentist may have a single helper who doubles as receptionist and dental assistant. When a dentist is his own boss, there are no other dentists to look over his shoulder to judge how he practices his profession. This dentist may be the best in the world. Or the worst.

Then how do you find a good dentist? If you intend to move to a new location, ask your present dentist or physician to recommend a competent dentist. When you're new in town, inquire at a dental school. Phone the local dental society, which will gladly refer you to qualified dentists. Ask your friends, co-workers, neighbors and other professionals whose opinions you respect to find out about their dentists. It is unwise to pick out a dentist blindly from the telephone book or go to a dentist who advertises: "no appointment necessary; extractions, dental plates in one day."

The best bet is a dental school if you're lucky enough to have one nearby. A dental school has a faculty made up of highly skilled dentists who are either professors or heads of various departments. Many of these dental teachers also have their own private practices. One phone call to the dental school, explaining your particular need, should put you in touch with an excellent dentist.

If you're not near a dental school, you might look in the telephone directory for a listing of the local dental society. The society will gladly recommend a good dentist. Or you might check in the directory for a specific dentist. Most list their practices after their names, such as "Practice Limited to Orthodontics," "Practice Limited to Endodontics," "Practice Limited to Periodontics," etc., and also "Member of ADA." That means they abide by the association's code of ethics.

Friends, neighbors and business associates may tell you they have a wonderful dentist. Maybe wonderful for them, but will the dentist be wonderful for you? Not necessarily, because no two people are alike and we all have individual needs. Do you require a dentist who can take care of the whole family—children, adults and older folks? Should your dentist be conveniently located so that you won't have to travel many miles to reach his office? Will you be able to make your dental appointments compatible with his office hours? Will you be happy going to the office of several dentists who practice as a group and where you may be scheduled to have Doctor A the first week and Doctor B the second week? Or the same situation in a dental clinic? Or do you prefer always to be treated by just one person?

Once you have decided to give a dentist a try, can you check on him before you make an appointment? Can you discuss your dental problems with him, ask about his qualifications, ask to see his credentials? Yes and no.

Whether you phone or go directly to his office, a good dentist's receptionist or dental assistant will readily describe the dentist's qualifications and credentials and explain that a complete oral examination would be required before the dentist could analyze your condition. A thorough examination with a set of full-mouth x rays, and sometimes casts, takes time—yours and the dentist's.

However, if you happen to have an emergency, most dentists would try to handle it if you can wait for him to find a free moment. Or his office may assist you in locating a dentist who can take care of the problem.

When you make an appointment, the receptionist should sound cheerful. She should explain the need for the oral examination, cleaning and scaling teeth, x rays and casts. She should also explain the dentist's fees for the procedures; if not, ask.

Look for diplomas and credentials on the walls of a dentist's office. There should be a diploma from an accredited dental school, other important credentials showing the dentist is a fellow of the American College of Dentists or a fellow of the

International College of Dentists. If he's a specialist, you should see the prized specialty board certification.

To practice a specialty is one thing. To be a board-certified specialist is another. In the USA, national specialty examining boards certify dentists who have put in two or three years of special graduate training and have passed exacting examinations. Only if he is board certified, or qualified and eligible to take the board, can a dentist legally call himself a specialist, one of a group of dedicated dentists who are generally considered the most reliable of all. However, many specialties have a "grandfather clause" allowing a dentist who graduated before a certain date to limit his practice to a specialty without having to take the special board examinations. There is also a cutoff date. For example, in endodontics, the "grandfather clause" permitted anyone who was graduated as a Doctor in Dental Surgery or Doctor of Dental Medicine before January 1965 to call himself a specialist and to practice endodontics without board certification and to have until January 1975 to prepare for board certification. After January 1975, all dentists wishing to limit their practice to endodontics must complete a 2 or 3-year graduate program to be qualified and eligible to take the certified board examination. There are eight specialties: orthodontics, periodontics, endodontics, oral surgery, oral pathology, pedodontics, prosthodontics and dental public health. We'll discuss all of them in later chapters.

Medical History

When you arrive for your first appointment, the receptionist or dental assistant will hand you a card asking for your medical history. A dentist needs this information so that he is aware of allergies to certain drugs, diabetes, high blood pressure or any other medical problem. Obviously this dentist is concerned with your total health, as well as your teeth, and properly so.

When a dentist asks for a medical history, it is not to diagnose or treat a patient's medical condition, but to evaluate it. He wants to know if the patient's physical health and emotional condition can tolerate a specific dental procedure. In case of doubt, the dentist will want to consult with the patient's physician. If a patient has a circulatory problem, diabetes, is a bleeder, is pregnant, is allergic to penicillin or other antibiotics and therapeutic agents, there may be possible risks. Here are some of the high-risk disorders you should be sure your dentist is aware of.

Diabetes. People with uncontrolled diabetes are poor candidates for withstanding dental stress and, in rare instances, may lapse into a coma. If, after questioning, the patient is doubtful about his condition and the diabetes appears to be uncontrolled, the dentist will want to consult with the patient's physician. Some diabetics have a tendency toward early development of arteriosclerosis.

Heart Failure. This is a not-uncommon hazard in a dental office. The patient's symptoms may include shortness of breath or swelling of the ankles. Heart patients usually take some form of digitalis, which should be reported to the dentist.

Angina Pectoris (extreme cardiac pain). The mortality rate of patients suffering from angina pectoris is 30 percent higher than average. The patient no doubt will be taking nitroglycerin to relieve the attack of pain, which may be precipitated by exertion or excitement. A wise dentist will work out a planned treatment with the patient's physician.

Coronary Occlusion. A patient with coronary occlusion also has a far greater mortality risk than the average. A person who has recovered from a coronary should be asked to supply a recent history and prognosis. Invariably, dentist and physician will hold a consultation before proceeding with any dental work.

Hypertension. This condition may lead to fainting or more serious troubles, such as a heart attack or a stroke. A detailed history should be given to the dentist. He will want to keep appointments short.

Blood Diseases. A patient with a history of leukemia, hemophilia or any hemorrhagic diseases should alert the dentist to consult the internist or hematologist. A report of previous bleeding experience or the use of anticoagulants warns the dentist to carry out preventive treatments to avoid any bleeding problems arising from surgery or other dental procedures.

Hyperthyroidism. A dentist will want to carefully evaluate anyone with a history of severe hyperthyroidism. Heart disease and angina pectoris may be related to the condition, which usually is accompanied by nervous actions, excessive perspiration and headaches.

Adrenal Insufficiency. If a patient takes cortisone or hydrocortisone, shock may occur during such minor treatments as a simple tooth extraction.

Certain drugs may entail definite risks for patients undergoing dental treatment. Countless individuals regularly take drugs prescribed by their physicians for various conditions; others are "on" drugs, an addictive habit. In either circumstance, the dentist must be aware of the patient's drug intake and any history of allergic reactions in order to avoid the administration of drugs which may cause toxic manifestations, erupting with catastrophic suddenness or emerging after long-term use. Some drugs are incompatible and may interfere with or increase the toxicity of the agents prescribed by the physician for other disorders. That is why an alert dentist will want to know if a patient is taking drugs and what they are.

Some of the commonly prescribed drugs a dentist looks for are chemical agents used to treat hypertension and hypotension; digitalis; nitroglycerin or anticoagulants; diuretics. Addictive use of analgesics (codeine, demerol), hypnotic drugs (barbiturates) tranquilizers or stimulants (amphetamines) can cause drug intoxication. One of the less dramatic manifestations of toxicity is the loss of sound judgment, which interferes with reasoning ability. This is one reason why dentists advise patients under sedation to have a relative or friend accompany them home.

A well-trained dentist is interested in protecting a patient. Many dentists insist on taking the blood pressure of any patient over the age of 15, especially if oral or intravenous sedation will be required. Most dentists and their assistants are prepared for emergencies. They keep on hand drugs to stop excessive bleeding, analgesics to relieve pain, spirits of ammonia to revive a patient who has fainted. Dentists and assistants know how to administer oxygen if needed and, in case of a heart attack, how to perform cardiopulmonary resuscitation (CPR).

X Rays

Your dentist depends on x rays to help him diagnose and treat conditions which might otherwise go undetected. Early decay, bone loss from gum disease, impacted teeth, abscesses, cysts and tumors are examples of conditions that are detected or confirmed by x-ray examination.

Dental x rays are a necessary part of comprehensive mouth care and, with the use of modern methods and equipment, they pose no threat to your health. The dentist and his staff have been trained to use minimum exposure. The amount of radiation you receive from dental x rays is less than that received from natural sources.

There are five types of x-ray pictures your dentist will need. The *periapical* x ray zooms in on one or two teeth, showing the entire tooth, including the apex of the root, and some of the surrounding tissues. *Bitewing* x rays provide a picture of upper and lower teeth on one film. A bitewing is especially useful in revealing small cavities and bone loss in the early stages of periodontal disease. An *occlusal* x ray shows the occlusal surfaces of the teeth and the dental arch and supplements periapical and bitewing x rays. These three types are called intraoral, because the film is held in the mouth when the picture is taken.

Extraoral x rays are used to show larger areas and the film is held outside the mouth. Extraorals are especially useful in spotting structural irregularities or unusual tissue growth, such as cysts or tumors. The *panoramic* x-ray machinery moves from one side of your jaw to the other. It provides a picture showing the upper and lower jaws, along with all teeth and other structures, in relationship to each other.

Examination and Diagnosis

When escorted to an examining room, it's a good idea to pause and take notice: is the room bright, cheerful and spotless? If the equipment is modern and well-kept, it's likely that the dentist is using the latest and best facilities and can give the best mechanical treatment.

After you have settled in the dental chair, the assistant should adjust the chair to make you comfortable, place a clean napkin around your neck and lay out sparkling, sterilized instruments on a spotless tray. A hygienist may clean and scale your teeth before you see the dentist. When you meet the dentist, is he friendly and interested in how and why you chose him? Does he ask about your present tooth problems and listen as you relate your dental history? After full-mouth x rays and a thorough scaling and cleaning of your teeth, the dentist will study the developed x rays and closely examine your teeth and gums. If you have no emergency problem, he may take impressions of your teeth and casts will be made so he can study the biting relationship of your teeth. Treatment plans will then be explained and discussed with you—it may be only one small filling or extensive work to save several ailing teeth. There's another clue: the dentist is talking about *saving* your teeth, not extracting them. Dentists who are quick to extract teeth probably don't know any other way to treat them or do not like to spend the time and effort to save them. Progressive dentists are strongly oriented toward preventive dentistry and saving of teeth. Modern dentistry, through well-devised treatment procedures, can save most teeth: the rare exception is a hopelessly broken down, nonrestorable tooth. If the circumstances of an individual case warrant it, a good general practitioner will refer his patient to a competent specialist.

After a complete oral examination, a good dentist will give you a specific, positive diagnosis. He will be confident and precise. He will explain why a procedure is necessary and discuss the alternatives with you. When you understand his proposal fully and you have confidence in him, you will usually be well advised to follow his advice.

While you're sizing him up, the good dentist will be sizing you up with probing questions. Do you clean your teeth diligently? How many times a day? How do you brush and how long? Do you smoke, drink alcohol? Do you have the habit of grinding your teeth? How did that fixed bridge get broken? He will talk in layman's language you can easily understand. He informs you about the fee—if not the precise amount, at least the range into which it will fall.

An experienced dentist will prepare you for changes in your mouth if you are about to have extensive restorations. If new appliances will bother you at first, the dentist will discuss the appliances and temporary discomfort. Knowing what's happening, why and how long it will last makes a patient feel a lot better.

Evaluating the Quality of Care

UNACCEPTABLE PROFESSIONAL STANDARDS

It isn't easy to recognize a dentist whose standards are low until you walk into his office, which is apt to be poorly equipped and untidy. Not that an elaborately equipped office is a guarantee of quality dentistry, but at least a good dentist has modern, well-functioning tools that can perform efficiently. Patients should be wary of assembly-line dentistry, when the dentist is rushing from chair to chair unable to give any patient enough time or care. Also, be aware of roughly finished fillings, shabbily contoured restorations and missing contact points, causing food impaction.

A discriminating patient can sense whether or not his dentist takes pride in his profession. Does he painstakingly carve and contour restorations, polish and shine amalgam fillings? Does he care about the patient's hygiene? Is he prevention minded, with a well-designed and well-organized plaque control program? Or is he extraction happy, pulling teeth at the slightest pain symptom because it is easier and faster to get rid of a problem tooth? Many wise patients who deserted their dentists express the following reasons: he fails to wash his hands before examining my mouth; his fingers smell of cigarettes; he never seems to be truly concerned about my teeth; he never explains what he's doing; he gets angry and defensive when I ask questions or suggest a consultation; he has bad breath and ugly-looking teeth—if he doesn't know how to take care of his dental problems, how can he take care of my mouth; he is grouchy, irritable and demeaning to his assistants.

Many people have left a longtime dentist because he is just

plodding along until retirement. They may have become genuinely fond of the man. He's almost a habit and anyone would feel pretty rotten deserting him. But if his dental equipment and his methods are outdated, he cannot possibly render the advantages of today's dental innovations and knowledge. It's unlikely, however, that there are many of these dear old souls around. Fortunately, most older dentists do take refresher courses and do keep up with current dentistry.

Actually, there are not too many dentists with substandard practices. The American dental profession is greatly concerned with maintaining its place as world leader in quality dental care and is making a renewed effort to police its membership by the creation of the Peer Review System. While the system evaluates dental care provided by dentists throughout America, the ADA is urging every state to require dentists and hygienists to show evidence of continuing education before renewing their licenses. And in order to protect the public from poor quality, illegal dentistry—particularly illegal denture work—by unqualified and untrained individuals, the ADA is suggesting periodic reexamination for members and mandatory continuing education.

A recent trend among local dental societies and state associations is the creation of a Peer Review. When a patient is not satisfied with a dentist's work, although the dentist may insist it was executed properly, the patient can appeal to the Peer Review and a patients-relation committee for recourse. If necessary, the committee will examine the dental work and make a recommendation to patient, dentist and, if one is involved, to the dental insurance plan. Dentists who are members of the ADA or local dental societies are obligated to abide by the decisions of the committee.

WORKING TOGETHER

You've found a great dentist when you can trust him, when you feel that you, the dentist, his receptionist, assistant and hygienist are all part of a family that works together with a common goal: *to obtain the best quality dental care available.* A lot depends also on you. You can be an ideal patient or a pain in the neck. The ideal patient is highly prevention minded; wants perfect dental health, not stop-gap repairs; faithfully visits the dental office every 6 months for professional maintenance. This patient is cooperative, is not nervous nor afraid and, when the work is completed, promptly pays the bill. Actually, the ideal patient takes such good care of his or her teeth that the dental bill is minimal.

Competent dentists understand patients' anxieties, feelings of self-pity, or habits of complaining. For example, an elderly gentleman arrived for his first appointment with a specialist and immediately related his past unhappy experiences. "I've had three sets of dentures made by three different dentists and none of them fit properly or looked natural," he said. "Someone recommended you, doc. I doubt if you can do any better than the others, but I'll give you a try."

"Please tell me about those dentures and why you didn't like them," suggested the experienced doctor as he sat down with the patient.

"First of all," the man confided, "no one can fit me correctly. Look! I have very small gums."

Interested, the dentist studied the man's mouth. "Yes, you do have small gums," he agreed as he began taking notes. In all sincerity, he added, "I believe that with special care I can fit you with dentures that will be reasonably snug and comfortable."

"If they're too tight, they'll hurt me."

"New dentures may hurt sometimes, but please don't worry. I will see to it that they won't hurt by adjusting them until they are comfortable."

"But what about the teeth? See these!" The man pointed to the front teeth. "They're too long, too dark, they don't match the others, and they don't look natural."

"I will do my best to make you a set of dentures looking so natural that it would be difficult to guess they're not your own teeth. We'll work together, you and I, until both of us are pleased."

The dentist carefully constructed the dentures, paying attention to all the patient's complaints. A few weeks later, having done the best he could, the dentist slipped the new dentures into his patient's mouth. The man was delighted with his improved appearance and comfort.

What was the dentist's secret? He had listened, he had cared, he had sympathized and he had paid close attention to the patient's grievances, whether real or imagined. As the dentist confides today, "I've learned that sometimes I must build dentures to fit the patient's head as well as his jaws."

Person-to-person communication often works wonders. And it works both ways. Your hard-working, conscientious dentist could use a little show of appreciation, especially after he has just saved a badly broken-down tooth or taken care of an emergency at 11 p.m. Dentists are human, too.

Sooner or later, your child will go to a dentist, usually about the age of two. It doesn't really make much difference whether the dentist is in general practice or is a pedodontist, so long as he is good. A young child, whose teeth have been well cared for, is not likely to have any major problems and there will be no time-consuming examination. The whole idea is to get the tot acquainted with the dental office, and give him an opportunity to learn to trust the dentist and understand that he will care for the small teeth. No drilling, nothing to frighten the child. Just fun. An experienced dentist knows how to inspire confidence in children and to work with them. He also knows how to relate to and work with parents.

Fees and Insurance

Every dentist sets his own fees, based on factors such as the time required and the complexity of each procedure. An ethical dentist will gladly tell you exactly what each procedure will cost, as well as any alternate program that he might recommend after a thorough study of your unique needs. Never feel embarrassed or afraid to ask, "How much will it cost?" You are the one who pays the bill and it's best to understand exactly what kind of treatment you are going to receive before you commit yourself. If a dentist says, "I'll make you a bridge. Come in next Thursday at three and we'll get started," it's your turn to ask, "What kind of bridge? A fixed bridge or a removable bridge? Is it to be made in gold,—gold and plastic or in gold and porcelain?"

A good dentist will take time to describe the type of bridge best suited. He will quote a fair price. If you come to him recommended by another trustworthy patient, he may not ask for a down payment, but he will—and rightfully—expect to be paid promptly when the work is completed. If the dentist knows you and your personal circumstances, he may occasionally allow you to pay in installments over a period of a few months. If costs are still more than you can handle, he may help you get a bank loan. A wise consumer will not proceed with dental work until the fee is clearly agreed upon.

Dental insurance is an up-and-coming factor. Recently, Californians paid over $1.2 billion for dental care, with insurance plans picking up over $200 million of the costs. Delta Dental Plans, operated by dentists as a nonprofit service corporation, is covering a percentage of dental fees in 47 states. Increasing numbers of trade unions, large and small companies, teachers' associations and other groups are offering dental insurance to their members or employees and their families. Insurance availability makes it easy for most patients to have needed dental work, permit more children to have their teeth straightened, more adults to get their teeth and gums in healthy condition and some older folks to wear comfortable dentures. With group insurance picking up an average of 50 to 80 percent of the dental fees, a member and his or her family can afford most dental work. If it is available to you in a group plan, you'll certainly want to take advantage of it. It may be well worth the high premium to enroll yourself in an individual program—but only you can decide.

5 TOOTH DECAY
When the drill is inevitable

Tooth decay is the most prevalent disease in the human race. Only 2 percent of the American population has been spared. Earliest cavities show up right after primary teeth erupt, most often starting in tiny fissures or pits. Tragically, tooth decay takes a tremendous toll on children; statistics reveal that the average 13-year-old already has five cavities in permanent teeth. Girls seem to get more cavities than boys, but then girls get their teeth sooner.

Why so many cavities? Perhaps because we have been inclined to take our teeth and gums for granted. Yet teeth and gums form an important part of that marvelous mechanism called the body. Dental and oral health can never be separated from general health and, if our general health is not the best, teeth and gums will bear the consequences. Malnutrition, some diseases and the effects of certain drugs will show up in our mouths. In fact, dentists often are the first to spot real medical problems.

Cavities and the Demon Plaque

CAUSES

A cavity is a hole in a tooth, caused by decay which is produced by plaque and acid. In the beginning it may be only a tiny hole, developing not only in pits and fissures, but wherever food collects. Day after day, the tiny hole will become deeper, softening and decalcifying the tooth enamel until it breaks through and spreads into the dentin. Then, every time you bite into a candy bar or drink a very cold or hot beverage you feel a sharp pain.

All the while, the cells of the pulp are trying to fight back by laying down fresh layers of dentin. If, however, the hole is widening and deepening faster than the fresh dentin can be replaced, decay and bacteria spread into the pulp. Soft pulp tissues, containing blood vessels and nerves, are exposed to all kinds of bacterial infection and inflammation.

Cavities, if not treated, can lead to toothache or a painful abscess. (If the toothache and abscess suddenly disappear without treatment, one should *not* consider the condition mysteriously cured. On the contrary, the pulp tissues have prematurely died and you have what laymen think of as a "dead tooth.")

Everyone except a newborn baby has countless numbers of bacteria swimming around and multiplying in his mouth. In fact, the new baby will start acquiring bacteria minutes after birth and the bacteria will remain with him the rest of his life.

These bacteria mix with saliva, shed epithelial cells (from gingiva and mucous linings of the oral cavity) and blood cells to form a thin, sticky, gelatin-like substance called *plaque.* Plaque clings tenaciously to the tooth surface and cannot be removed by rinsing or water spray. It is now generally accepted that even if the bacteria which cause dental decay or periodontal disease are present in the mouth, they cannot cause disease until they are attached to the teeth as a component of plaque. Evidence today points to bacteria amassed in the plaque as the

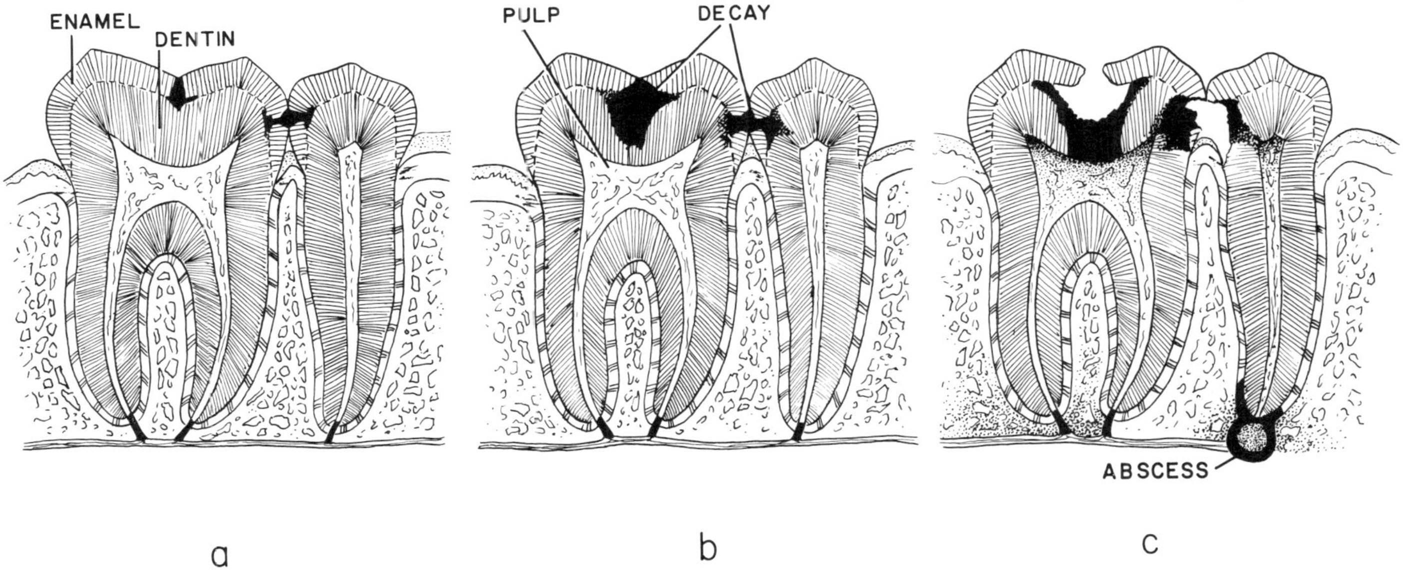

Tooth decay. (a) A small cavity in the enamel, left untreated, enlarges and attacks the dentin. (b) Decay spreads, approaching the pulp. (c) Decay invades the pulp and bacteria travel through the pulp cavity. Finally, an abscess forms around the root tip.

primary agents in producing dental decay and periodontal disease.

Plaque will cling to the vulnerable parts of the teeth: all areas except the flat biting surfaces and sides where the tongue or cheeks are constantly producing a cleaning action. Harmful bacteria also creep around the gums. Once bacteria have dug into a spot on a tooth, above or below the gum margin, a colony of bacteria moves in. Within a few days, they will increase their population tremendously and become more complex; plaque will thicken.

But it doesn't take a few days for trouble to develop. Tooth decay can start in less than 15 minutes after eating. All that is needed are three ingredients: a tooth, bacteria and sugar. When bacteria and sugar meet, acid is formed. And when acid and tooth meet, the acid starts etching a little hole in the tooth enamel, the protective armor. The more sugar you eat, the more acid you will have in your mouth. The more acid, the more etching of enamel. As enamel becomes weakened and eroded, bacteria break through, eat the dentin and bore into the pulp: a cavity results.

TYPES

There are several varieties of cavities, *pit* and *fissure* being the most common. These are protected niches where bacteria can develop undisturbed. A greater number of bacteria swarm into the pits and fissures than into any other parts of a tooth and, for that reason, earliest cavities are likely to be in these places.

Then there are the *smooth-surface* cavities. They occur frequently between two teeth where food and bacteria have been allowed to collect and they are difficult to detect without x rays. A smooth-surface cavity is rarely found on the exposed front or back of a tooth, because these surfaces are automatically cleaned during chewing and are easy to brush.

Third are *gumline cavities,* which occur as you get older, your gums recede and plaque is allowed to build around the necks of teeth. Fourth are *root cavities,* observed in older persons who neglect mouth hygiene to such an extent that recession of the gums exposes the root. Since the root is covered only by cementum, it is much softer than enamel and an easy prey to bacteria. Both gumline cavities and root cavities result from poor brushing and a diet high in carbohydrates.

PREVENTION

How can we prevent cavities? Four ways: fluoridation, correct diet, proper dental hygiene to remove bacterial dental plaque, regular checkups.

Fluoride's greatest benefits are seen with children's teeth, especially in an area where natural fluoridation exists in the drinking water. To prevent mottling of enamel by excess fluoride, this water must be filtered to contain an optimum amount of fluoride—about 1 to 1½ parts per 1 million parts of water.

But how about artificial fluoridation? Success again. After experiments in which 1 part of fluoride added to 1 million parts of drinking water proved teeth would not become discolored, controlled artificial fluoridation became a way of life in many of our states. Scientists watched carefully and, in due time, their studies showed a 55 to 60 percent reduction in the number of decayed teeth, lost teeth and filled teeth in children who had been drinking the artificially fluoridated water since birth.

In the United States, questions about fluoridation started almost 80 years ago when dentists became interested in the brown stain on the teeth of individuals living in El Paso, Colorado. By 1931, it was decided that fluoride was the chemical in the water that caused this stain. They named it Colorado Brown Stain and now refer to it as *mottled enamel* or *enamel fluorosis.* After further studies, scientists concluded that individuals who had been drinking fluoridated water all their lives had fewer cavities than the population at large. And that's why many communities began adding fluoride to the water supply: more than 70 percent of our population is now drinking either naturally or artifically fluoridated water.

Proper diet is vital to dental health. What we eat and drink will definitely determine the life of our teeth. To have a mouthful of cavities and, eventually, no teeth at all, just eat lots of sweet desserts, drink lots of sugared soda pops, and forget to brush and floss your teeth.

Sugar—refined, powedered, brown, raw or called by any other name—is still sugar and it is the stuff that causes decay: frequently, quickly and efficiently. The average American consumes about 115 pounds of sugar a year, or one teaspoonful every 30 minutes.

Consider the average daily sugar intake of all too many children: sugar-coated cereal and more sugar added from the sugar bowl; sugar-sweetened chewing gum; a jelly doughnut and a sugar-sweetened cola drink; ice cream, cookies and more sugared gum; sugar-sweetened canned fruit in salad, candied yams, cake with frosting; candy bars.

Not only is this a tremendous amount of sugar, but it is sugar that is taken into the mouth all day long and never brushed or flossed away. At least, not until bedtime. Think of all the sugar that is accumulating on your children's teeth (maybe your teeth, too?) and how the bacteria are having a picnic forming acid, while the acid is etching and melting away tooth enamel.

Can we change the picture? Yes, but don't expect fluoridated water alone to stop the ravages caused by a poor diet. A proper diet is certainly necessary and that doesn't mean popping a few vitamin tablets and telling yourself they will take care of the problem. They won't. The stickier the food, the more likely it is to adhere to the teeth. It would be wiser to eat detergent foods, rough, tough materials which we must heartily chew, food that will not stick to our teeth. Detergent foods actually help clean teeth and stimulate the gums. Raw celery and raw carrots are examples.

The most important tooth saver of all is yourself and your home care. That means using good toothbrushes, a dentrifrice, dental floss, a water irrigating unit and time set aside every day to fight the battle against tooth decay.

Understandably, you can't brush, floss and flush when you are eating out. You can, however, reduce the germ and bacteria concentration and remove a great deal of food debris by placing a small amount of water, tea or coffee in your mouth and forcefully moving this liquid around your teeth. This "swish and swallow" procedure repeated four or five times immediately after eating has proved to be an effective method of eliminating retained material from the mouth. Anything you can do to remove food debris will help prevent decay and gum disease.

Everyone should see his dentist twice a year. He can catch a small decay before it becomes a major problem. Approximately 45 percent of American youngsters under the age of 15 have never visited a dentist nor had a dental examination. Moreover, it is quite possible that as many as one billion unfilled and decayed teeth are in the mouths of our citizens at this very moment.

Without a doubt, there will be some readers who will say, "But how come my grandfather, who died at the age of 85, had all of his teeth and no cavities?"

A good question, indeed. And here's the answer.

If your grandfather lived to be 85 without a cavity, he probably had a special ingredient in his saliva, a protein dentists call *secretory immunoglobulin A.* This protein seems to fight off bacteria by coating or altering the bad bacteria so that they can't form acids that start tooth decay. If tests had been made of grandfather's saliva, they most likely would have shown that he had a very high concentration of antibacterial agents. Therefore, he could even eat sweets, forget to brush his teeth and still remain cavity-free. Of course, we suspect he didn't eat much refined sugar, either.

What are your chances? And what are your children's chances? Remember, only 2 percent of our population gets away without tooth decay. Now you know what causes decay and how to prevent it. Reread Chapter 3, which details the benefits of fluoridation, proper nutrition, and the importance of a thorough daily hygienic routine. If you follow it faithfully, you may never need to face the dentist's drill.

Locating and Classifying Cavities

THE PRELIMINARIES

Most of us have experienced the dentist's drill, but very few of us really understood what was going on.

Suppose your lower left first molar becomes sensitive to sweets or to cold or hot liquids. You suspect a cavity and make a dental appointment. In the dental chair, you tell the dentist which tooth hurts, how long a time it has been bothering you and whether the pain is steady or intermittent.

First, the dentist wants an x ray which will reveal whether or not there actually is decay and, if so, where, how far and how deep, how close to the nerve. Is the cavity situated in the front surface, the back surface, between the teeth? Is there an infection, an abscess? All of these things cannot be accurately detected by the dentist merely examining a tooth with his explorer.

Some people are afraid of x rays because of exposure to radiation. The early x-ray machines required long exposures and there were certain dangers. Today, however, a dentist's diagnostic x ray is taken in a split second. In fact, it gives off an extremely low dosage of radiation compared to such high-dose examinations as a gastrointestinal series or a spinal examination.

Complete or *full-mouth x rays* every two or three years and *bitewing* x rays once a year are sufficient for the average patient. All ethical dentists will provide a patient with a lead apron to cover the body from chin to thighs as a precaution against radiation.

Without an x ray of a sick tooth, your dentist would be groping in the dark. He could be unaware of an infection in the root, tartar below the gumline or decay under an old filling. With an x ray, your dentist has a complete picture of the tooth, an accurate guide on where to drill, how wide and how deep.

Most dentists display a patient's x rays by clipping them onto a viewer. Ask your dentist to explain your x rays: how a decayed area shows as a dark shadow, the number of fillings, the nerves, the roots, how an impacted wisdom tooth looks.

CLASSES OF CAVITIES

When a cavity shows up in that lower left molar, the first question is what part of the tooth it is located in. The side facing the cheek is the *buccal* surface; the side facing the tongue is called the *lingual* surface; the *distal* surface is most distant from the median line and the *mesial* surface is closest to the median line; *occlusal* means on the chewing surface and *proximal* means between two teeth. A cavity occurring on only one surface is a simple cavity; if it occurs on two or more surfaces, it is a compound cavity.

How a cavity will be treated depends on which tooth is in trouble. Six main types of cavities exist and each one requires individual consideration.

Class I includes molars which have cavities on the chewing surfaces or on the buccal or lingual surfaces. Class I also includes upper incisors which have cavities on the lingual surfaces.

All other classes are considered smooth-surface cavities.

Class II indicates cavities on proximal surfaces of molars and bicuspids, usually with two or more surfaces involved.

Class III refers to cavities on the proximal surfaces of incisors and canines.

Class IV includes cavities on the proximal surfaces of incisors and canines, extending to the cutting edge of the tooth and requiring the removal and restoration of the incisal angle.

Class V designates cavities in the gingival area of the labial, buccal and lingual surfaces (including pit cavities).

Class VI refers to cavities occuring on the incisal edges or on the tips of the cusps.

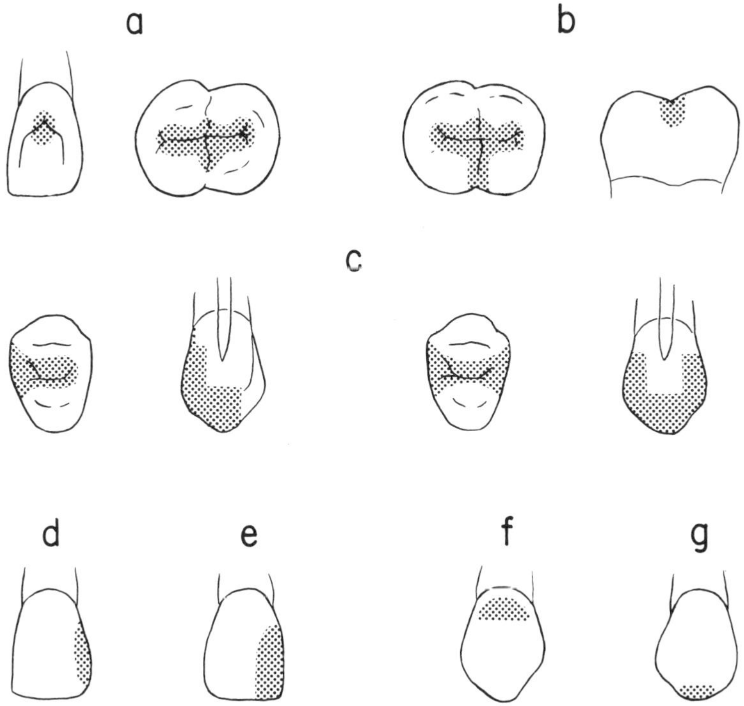

Classification of cavities. (a) Simple Class I. (b) Compound Class I. (c) Class II. (d) Class III. (e) Class IV. (f) Class V. (g) Class VI.

Filling Materials

Assuming that yours is a simple Class I cavity, the next step is to consider the filling. You and your dentist will discuss the matter before the drilling starts because different filling materials call for different drilling patterns.

If a filling is going to show when you smile, porcelain will be the answer—*if* the filling is not a large one. For the record, a porcelain filling really won't be porcelain, it will only look that way. In the past, a refined cement powder named silicate was popular, but because this filling material discolored and washed out in time, better materials took its place. New tooth-colored materials are called composite filling materials. These contain various reinforcing agents, such as quartz crystals or glass particles, to improve wearing strength, durability and resistance to color changes. These materials can be cleverly matched to the color of your own teeth.

The most popular filling material is amalgam, often called a "silver" filling. But that's a misnomer. Silver fillings are actually produced from an alloy of mercury, tin, copper and sometimes zinc, together with 65 to 75 percent of silver powder. After the dentist has cleaned and lined your tooth cavity, he will mix this amalgam and pack it into the hole. When the cavity is filled, the dentist carves the amalgam to conform to the shape and contour of the tooth. He checks your bite and carves a little more in case it is still too high.

If a cavity is a large one, an *inlay* may be in order, usually in gold. First, a dentist prepares the cavity so that he can take a perfect wax impression. An inlay requires parallel and slightly diverging walls, free from undercuts, so the gold casting can be inserted and withdrawn while checking the fit. While waiting for the dentist or the laboratory to make the gold inlay, the patient will have a temporary cement filling. When the gold inlay is ready, the dentist removes the temporary and tests the fitting of the inlay, checking to be sure the bite is comfortable. He then cements the gold inlay in place and polishes it. A good gold inlay usually lasts for many years and is considered stronger than a good amalgam filling.

Sometimes a single tooth has several cavities and filling it is impossible. The solution is a crown. A *crown* can be made of porcelain, gold covered by porcelain, or gold, and it looks like a tight-fitting cap. In fact, a crown is also called a cap or a jacket. When the dentist has cleaned out a cavity and reduced the height and circumference of the tooth so that it can receive a crown, he takes an impression with one of a variety of rubber-like or latex materials.

Dental lab technicians build the new crown according to specifications: perhaps an all-metal crown for a back tooth or a porcelain-bonded-to-gold crown for a front tooth. When the dentist receives the completed crown, he cements it over the prepared tooth and the patient has a beautiful new tooth which should serve him well.

Cost, of course, is a factor. Amalgam is the least expensive; next are the composite resins. Gold foil follows. The most expensive would be the gold inlay, taking into consideration rising prices for gold, lab work and the dentist's extra time. It's a good idea to ask the dentist what each type of filling will cost and how he wants you to pay so that arrangements are understood before work begins.

Drilling and Filling

Once the material is decided upon, the dentist will make preparations to shape the cavity correctly and safely to accommodate the filling. Let's say you decided on an amalgam filling. You are reclining in the dental chair with the dentist on one side and the dental assistant on the other. The treatment begins with the administration of anesthetic to prevent pain. First, a topical anesthetic (usually an ointment) is placed on the gum area where the dentist will inject a local anesthetic. Xylocaine is the most widely used local anesthetic today (Novocain and procaine have not been in wide use for many years; Xylocaine has far fewer side effects). The needle is eased into the gum and there's a smarting sensation, similar to a small cut on your finger. In one or two minutes, the anesthetic has taken effect.

Now treatment begins. A rubber dam may be stretched over the lower part of your face. A rubber dam is a square sheet of rubber with holes fitted tightly around several teeth, including the tooth to be treated. The tooth will remain dry. When the dentist works with the rubber dam it is called a "dry field." However, with a simple Class I cavity, you are more likely to receive cotton rolls and a saliva ejector in your mouth.

The dentist probably will start to work with a high-speed water-cooled air drill, a grinding tool technically called an air-turbine handpiece. Later, he may switch to a slower, belt-driven or air-driven drill which offers him more control for the finer touches of cavity preparation. Burs are the small drills placed in the tip of the dental handpiece. They are made of carbide steel or bonded diamond particles on a steel shank; some are used for drilling, others for polishing. If you find the drilling loud, it is because your mouth becomes an echo chamber; vibrations from the drill are conducted directly to your ears through the jawbone.

Before you know it, the drill penetrates the enamel and reaches the decay area in the dentin. But the job is far from over. Further drilling is needed as the dentist extends the cavity outline. Retention forms and undercuts are made to be sure the filling will withstand the stress of chewing and not fall out with the first tug of a sticky caramel.

In four-hand dentistry (dentist and dental assistant), the assistant busily evacuates saliva, water spray and drilling debris with a powerful suction mechanism. Finally, the dentist, using a spoon-shaped instrument called an excavator, will carefully scoop out all decayed dentin, then flush the cavity with more streams of water and air until absolutely no decay is left.

But how can a dentist know positively that he has removed all the decay, especially when the cavity is close to the nerve? He can dig too far and risk injuring the nerve, or he can dig too little, and inadvertently not remove all decay. If decay remains, it will spread and, left unattended, the nerve may die and root canal treatment would be needed to save the tooth. However, there are ways of knowing when all decay is gone. Decay is a soft, mushlike substance. When the excavator sinks into soft matter, the dentist knows there is still decay in the cavity. When he reaches sound dentin, he will recognize a distinctive sound, the "dentinal cry," and can be sure he has removed all the decay.

With the molar now as clean as a whistle, the tooth is ready for the amalgam filling. How will it be applied? Because the cavity is not too deep, the tooth will not require an insulation of cement base or a coat of varnish used in deep-seated cavities. Your cavity will be kept dry while the dental assistant mixes the amalgam and passes it to the dentist in an amalgam carrier. The dentist discharges the amalgam into the cavity and, using small pluggers, condenses the amalgam into the cavity.

A few minutes later, as the amalgam begins to harden slightly, the dentist, using carving instruments, carves the amalgam into proper anatomical form. The dentist will check your bite by inserting a carbonlike paper between the molars and asking you to bite gently. A blue carbon mark left on the filling will tell if there is a high spot that must be carved down. When the bite is perfect, the dentist will dismiss you. But if he's conscientious, he will polish your amalgam filling at a later date. Normally, you can eat an hour after leaving the office. The anesthetic also should wear off within an hour.

More complex cavities may require a variation in this routine. Basically, a filling can have one, two, three or more surfaces. A one-surface filling means the walls of the tooth are strong and healthy and can surround and support a filling. A one-surface filling can be anywhere—on the chewing surface, on the buccal or the lingual surface. A two-surface filling could involve replacing the chewing surface and one side of the tooth. A three-surface filling might be the same, except that the filling would extend to a second side of the tooth.

The amount of work and time required for an appointment is based on the number of surfaces requiring restoration, plus the condition of the tooth. If the cavity is close to the nerve, extra care must be taken. If the cavity is so deep that it is very close to the pulp, it will be lined with pulp-protecting material, such as ZNOE, a compound of zinc oxide and eugenol that smells like oil of cloves. If a healthy pulp is exposed, the dentist sometimes can successfully cap the pulp without resorting to root canal treatment.

You may wonder how anyone could get a cavity deep enough to reach the pulp. The answer is one word: *neglect.* If the pulp capping should fail, there will most likely be pain. To save the tooth would then require root canal treatment, which is discussed in Chapter 7.

CONTOURING AND FINISHING FILLINGS

Contouring and finishing fillings can make or ruin a tooth and its supporting structures. Fillings involving the sides of two adjoining teeth must be contoured correctly so that both contact points of the teeth meet tightly. Contact points are tested with dental floss. If the floss slips through the contacts with room to spare, the new filling may be undercontoured, its sides straight instead of fully contoured. Weak contacts allow food to pack between the teeth, resulting in irritation and periodontal problems. If new fillings allow food packing, ask to have the fillings changed and contoured properly.

A two-surface or three-surface filling requires the use of a matrix around the tooth while the filling is being condensed. The matrix is a steel band, if the dentist is using amalgam. It can be a celluloid strip help tightly by the dentist if the filling is a composite material. The purpose of the celluloid strip is to give good form and contour to the filling by preventing the material from spilling over the margins. The matrix also keeps the filling in shape as it hardens.

An inlay is prepared much the same as any other cavity, with two exceptions. An inlay needs an occlusal dovetail to lock the inlay securely in place and prevent it from rocking itself loose. Also, the walls of the cavity are slightly divergent occlusally to allow for withdrawal and insertion of the gold inlay. When the cavity is completely clean and well prepared, an impression is made. The impression is sent to a dental laboratory that will make the inlay or the dentist himself may make it.

The dentist will test the new inlay in the tooth, perhaps grinding off a tiny bit here or there to obtain a perfect fit. When it's satisfactory, the dentist will cement the inlay in place. Then follows the bite test, the final polishing and it's all over.

An onlay is similar to an inlay, although it is larger, covering two or more sides of the tooth and the chewing surface. An onlay is made in the same manner as an inlay, but it will cost more.

Gumline cavities (caused only by poor hygiene) call for a different treatment. Sometimes they are not simply gumline cavities, they are cavities below the gum margin which must be handled with care. A gumline cavity, after the usual drilling, can be filled with amalgam, a composite or gold foil. The very best that dentistry can offer is gold foil for gumline cavities that don't show. Today, however, dentistry is cosmetically minded and the tendency is to avoid shining metal in the mouth. Thus, the so-called porcelain filling has become more desirable and is used more frequently.

If your tooth has a large amalgam filling and has been filled many times in the past, one more patching job may not be wise nor practical. The dentist will examine the tooth and, if the old fillings appear insecure, he will remove them entirely, together with the decay. As the tooth is broken down, it must be built up again before a crown preparation can be made. Amalgam or composite filling and pins will be used for this reconstruction. Then the tooth is slightly reduced to complete the crown preparation.

An impression is made of the preparation. The crown can be made in gold, or porcelain bonded to gold. The crown will be tested, fitted, adjusted, and contoured to correct anatomical form. The dentist will check contacts and bite, and will polish the crown before cementing it onto the tooth. A well-made crown gives excellent protection for many years.

Erosion and Abrasion

Erosion is abnormal wear of a tooth resulting in smooth, notched-out depressions, especially on the facial surfaces near the gumline. The causes of erosion are believed to be primarily chemical. The habit of sucking lemons, for example, can dissolve tooth enamel and dentin.

Abrasion is the wearing away of tooth structure by mechanical means. It can be caused by brushing teeth sideways instead of in the direction that the teeth grow. Teeth are often abraded because of pencil and pen-biting, hairpin or nail-holding habits.

Eroded and abraded areas often need to be filled. The dentist may make a regular cavity preparation and fill it with amalgam, gold foil or composite material. These days, he can also fill many eroded areas without cutting into the tooth by using the *acid-etched method.* The dentist applies an acid solution to the clean, dry surface of the enamel. The acid is washed off with water and the tooth is dried with air. He then applies the bonded restorative material to the tooth area that has been etched. Application of the composite material can be made by brushing, painting, packing and shaping with instruments.

Ultraviolet light helps to set the material. Results with the new restorative materials have been promising and repairs have held up well in a majority of cases. However, this bonding technique will not work at all if it is applied to dentin. It must only be bonded to enamel.

In all dentist-patient relationships there can be deficiencies, oversights and poor judgment. If a new filling doesn't seem right, go back to the dentist and explain. Frequently there is a valid reason for a shortcoming. Perhaps a tiny piece of filling chipped off or maybe the gum was bleeding slightly and the dentist was unable to see the excess filling.

Whatever the cause, a conscientious dentist wants you to return and voice your complaint. He has done his best and, if something has gone wrong, he is anxious to correct it. Don't air your complaints to a friend, mother or neighbor. These people can't help. The dentist can.

6 PERIODONTICS
The treatment of gum diseases

Periodontal disease is curable and teeth can be saved if you do not let the disease progress. Too often, patients go to the dentist only when they have pain or when they recognize that something has gone wrong. Waiting is an expensive game, for periodontists have been around a long time, ready to treat and heal.

Periodontal disease is the major cause of tooth loss for three out of four adults aged 40 or older, but children are not exempt. According to statistics, 95 percent of children 5 to 14 years old have some degree of gum inflammation and one out of four has some loss of gum attachment around the teeth.

Periodontal disease is a severe inflammation of the gums due to a buildup of plaque and tartar; the result is destruction to the supporting tissues around your teeth. This destruction includes: your gums; the periodontal fibers or ligaments that hold your teeth in your jaws; cementum, the bony substance that covers the roots of your teeth; and alveolar bone that supports each tooth socket.

Originally, our gums were perfectly formed but, with the

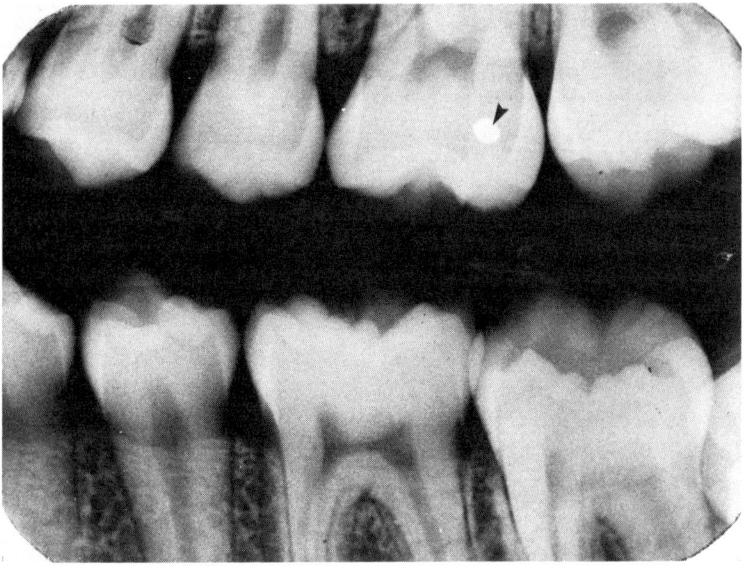

An almost perfect set of teeth, free from decay, show up on this bitewing x ray of the left side of a 22-year-old's mouth. Arrow indicates a small amalgam filling.

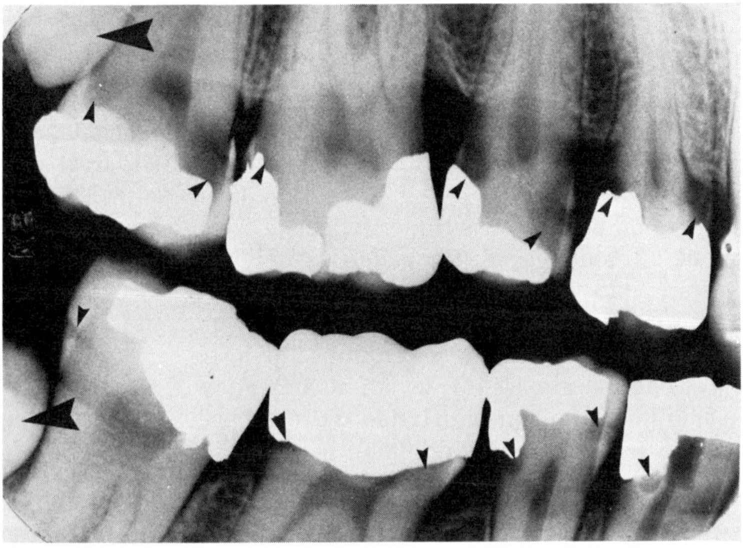

Numerous restorations (white areas) and a great number of cavities (dark shadow areas at arrows) show up on this bitewing x ray of a 27-year-old mouth. Large arrows indicate impacted wisdom teeth.

development of periodontal disease, gums change color, texture and shape and teeth begin to feel loose even in early stages. Form and function become changed. As bacterial plaque spreads below the gums into the periodontal tissues, the tissues become affected and teeth become wobbly. The dentist can reverse the condition by conscientiously scaling and cleaning plaque and tartar from the teeth. Only when all plaque and tartar are completely removed will the gums regain their elasticity and return to normal appearance. Teeth will then become firm again.

Normally, our teeth move slightly when we chew. If your teeth were set solidly in your jaw, they would break almost every time you bit into a hard roll. Teeth are attached to bone by ligaments that constantly are in action, giving and taking as you chew. With periodontal disease, teeth move more than usual, membranes around the teeth are likely to deteriorate and toxic substances may get into the blood stream.

If disease is not treated and cured in its early stages, gums begin to separate from the teeth. The resulting spaces between gums and teeth fill up—as unpleasant as seems—with plaque, tartar, bacteria and pus. The disease goes on to attack the bone that cradles the teeth until the bone is destroyed, leaving teeth with nothing to hold them. Teeth then may become so loose they either fall out or must be extracted. However, teeth will never suffer from periodontal disease unless plaque and tartar are allowed to form.

Fortunately, dentistry has the knowledge to prevent or retard the development of periodontal disease and to treat those afflicted. Periodontology is the specialty concerned with the study and treatment of diseases and structures that support the bone, ligaments, and roots; a periodontist is the specialist who treats periodontal disease.

Gingival Diseases

GINGIVITIS

The earliest stage of gum disease is *simple gingivitis,* an inflammation of the tissue. With dental mirror in hand, you can check for the indications. The first sign of gingivitis is when you notice that the tips of the gingiva triangles between teeth are losing their healthy pink color, seem to be swollen, are slightly red and slightly curled. The triangles no longer form firm peaks. The gums bleed easily.

Advanced gingivitis will signal its presence with blood on your toothbrush. Close inspection will reveal gum irritation, inflammation and the beginning of detachment of the gum margins. Plaque and food are now able to slip between gingiva and tooth. Gums are swollen and may feel tender or sore. This kind of detachment of gingiva, however, is not the same as the recession or erosion of teeth.

Very young children are not as likely to have gingivitis as teenagers and adults. First of all, the young are healthy and haven't had time to build up bacteria. Secondly, their teeth are not inclined to be as crowded as are those of adults and they can be cleaned more easily. Also, they don't have the fillings and bridgework of adults, which often catch debris. But gingivitis does appear when young children fail to brush their teeth correctly on a daily schedule. Parents of very young children should either brush them or, better still, begin supervising them in correct brushing and flossing. Problems begin when children start wearing orthodontic bands without increasing their brushing time. Gingivitis is not limited to adults. It bears repeating that 95 percent of children ages 5 to 15 already have some degree of gum trouble.

PYORRHEA

Another form of advanced gum disease, known as *pyorrhea* or *periodontitis,* is a severe inflammation which causes the gums to fall away from the necks of the teeth. Large amounts of plaque, food and tartar are increasingly invading the gingival crevices, causing increased irritation. The more irritation, the more the gums seem to withdraw from the source of irritation (plaque and tartar). As the detachment of gums continues, the bones underneath the gums start to resorb or dissolve and some teeth will begin to feel loose. Deep gum pockets are present here and there. Pressing gently on the gum margin is likely to reveal pus. Gums will bleed more profusely and breath will not be very pleasant.

In *advanced periodontitis,* the teeth appear longer because the gum line has receded and fallen away, revealing the roots of the teeth. In some places, as much as half of the gingival coverage may have been lost and the teeth are sitting in very little bone. The gum is no longer snug, but fits the tooth like an old rubber band. If one tooth or many teeth are loose, one should seek dental treatment immediately.

PERIODONTOSIS

A rare form of periodontal disease seen in young people, frequently in women, is known as *periodontosis.* It is characterized by early loosening and migration of teeth. The first permanent molars and incisors are most often involved, with severe bone loss. This disease seems to be caused by the degeneration and inflammation of the periodontal tissues.

PREGNANCY GINGIVITIS

Pregnant women often suffer gum swelling without realizing why. A young woman finally visited her dentist during the last two months of pregnancy with her gums so inflamed and swollen that they almost completely covered her teeth. She had no idea that such a condition as *pregnancy gingivitis* existed and consequently was at a loss to understand what was happening to her. She kept waiting for the condition to clear up. Instead, it got worse, for she had procrastinated much too long.

Every pregnant woman should know what pregnancy gingivitis is and be able to recognize it in her own mouth. She should follow a stringent oral hygiene program, regularly examining her mouth, and have her teeth cleaned professionally, once at the beginning of pregnancy and again near the end. If she has any doubts, she should check with her dentist or visit a dental clinic at once instead of waiting until after the baby is born. Good hygiene is a preventive as well as a treatment. Increased home and professional dental care can prevent this variety of gingivitis.

TRENCH MOUTH

Everyone should watch out for trench mouth, so named because soldiers in World War I who fought in trenches were afflicted by this serious gum disease. In those days, trench mouth was believed to be passed from soldier to soldier via dirty canteens or dirty dishes, or caught by kissing someone who was already infected. Later, the dental profession named trench mouth *necrotizing ulcerative gingivitis* or *Vincent's infection* and declared that the condition is, in fact, rarely infectious. World War I soldiers did not get trench mouth from dirty utensils or kissing. They got it from lack of proper oral hygiene, from stress and poor nutrition.

Can anyone get trench mouth? Yes, indeed. Anyone—with or without teeth—can come down with this very unpleasant, uncomfortable gum disease. But it is easy to recognize. Recall the symptoms of ailing gums discussed under gingivitis and pyorrhea: the loss of healthy pink color, the swelling, the bleeding, the gums falling away from the teeth. Add to that the unique symptoms of trench mouth.

Trench mouth can strike suddenly, afflicting all teeth and gums. Gums will bleed quite freely. Upon inspection of the mouth with a mirror, you will notice that the centers of those triangular gingival peaks between teeth have more or less collapsed, looking like craters in a tiny volcano. There is a gray membrane covering the gums. There may be a metallic taste in the mouth. Breath odor will be repulsive and one may have a headache and low-grade fever.

The gums will hurt, especially when you scrape off the gray membrane, which can happen quite readily with a toothbrush. But then the gums bleed and later the gray membrane returns. Actually, the brush is taking off the top of an infected wound. Symptoms may sound frightening, but trench mouth can be cured quickly and easily.

What causes trench mouth? Well, for many years the dental profession was puzzled and only recently have experts gone along with the theory that certain oral microorganisms can bring on the condition. Those microorganisms can attack the mouth only if you do not get enough sleep, do not eat a well-balanced diet, overindulge in alcohol consumption, smoke too much, and particularly if you fail to keep your mouth clean.

Trench mouth can be serious, but your dentist and you have the knowledge and equipment required to cure the trouble. The first move is yours. See your dentist on an emergency basis. If you have to wait for an appointment, start immediately on a home treatment program. Rinse your mouth with warm salt water (as warm as you can stand) for 4 or 5 minutes every hour. Use a level teaspoonful in a large glass of warm water. In addition, use 3 percent hydrogen peroxide—available at any drugstore—as a mouthwash 2 or 3 times a day. Take large doses of vitamin C tablets, 1200 to 1500 milligrams daily depending on your body weight, for the duration of the disease.

Eat a lot of fresh vegetables and fruits rich in Vitamin C. Avoid irritating and highly seasoned foods. Above all, brush your gums and teeth 5 or 6 times a day with a medium-soft toothbrush. Yes! Even if it hurts and bleeds. The more the gums bleed, the more often you should brush.

If you are lucky enough to see your dentist at once, you probably will be given antibiotics. Teeth will be scaled to remove the worst of the deposits along the gumline. Three or four days later, using an anesthetic, the dentist will scale *under* the gumline. A third visit may be the final scaling for awhile. Teeth will be polished and you will be sent home to carry out a prescribed routine of oral hygiene.

Causes and Prevention

SMOKING, ALCOHOL AND DRUGS

Not all gum problems are due to the lack of sensible oral hygiene. For example, the drug Dilantin is successful in controlling epilepsy, but the drug takes its toll on the gingiva. Those individuals using Dilantin find their gums swelling as though infected. If the gums are already irritated and inflamed from lack of good dental care, the swelling will increase. Unfortunately, there is no way of stopping the swelling caused by Dilantin itself, but anyone who is taking the drug is well advised to keep his or her teeth and gums in top shape.

Smoking, excessive drinking of alcohol, and using drugs

such as Methedrine, Dexedrine, cocaine, etc., tend to adversely affect the gums. The elimination of many drugs is carried through the tissues of the oral cavity.

Excessive consumption of alcoholic beverages and indiscriminate use of oral antiseptics tend to dry and burn the oral mucous membranes. Cells in the mouth may die. There is also a sudden imbalance of microorganisms in the mouth for a short time. This condition allows harmful bacteria to multiply and take over.

It is known that heavy smoking diminishes local vascular accessibility and blood flow. This is due to the vasoconstrictive effect of nicotine, which causes a relative tissue ischemia (localized tissue anemia due to obstruction of the inflow of arterial blood). In addition, the deposits of nicotine stains on the teeth tend to encourage plaque formation.

Heavy smoking frequently affects the oral mucosa in an adverse manner. For instance, there was a man who smoked two to three packs of cigarettes daily. One day, the dentist noticed white plaque on the man's cheeks, palate and gums. He let the patient see these areas of irritation and tissue changes under a good light.

"We call those white patches leukoplakia and they could become malignant," said the dentist. "Why don't you try to stop smoking?"

To impress the patient with the unwanted changes in his oral tissues, the dentist took impressions of the patient's mouth and poured stone casts of the impressions. Roughness and a leathery, cracked-tissue pattern were evident on the stone cast. "If you will stop smoking at least four weeks, I'm sure your oral tissues will look much better," the dentist said. Four weeks later, another set of impressions were taken. The surface texture of the tissue appeared smoother, not cracked, not leathery. The patient's mouth looked healthier and nearly normal again. The patient was so impressed by the startling difference that he never smoked again.

PLAQUE

If you brush and floss meticulously enough to remove entirely all trace of plaque from all teeth, you're on the right track. Once plaque is removed, it takes the bacteria 24 hours to reorganize into plaque and attach to the tooth surfaces again.

For the average person, however, brushing and flossing thoroughly after every meal has proved to be more beneficial. If plaque is the villain, we should try to destroy it in every way possible. Don't forget your diet plan. No sugar. Sugar in your mouth turns into acid, which attacks the tooth enamel. Other foods, such as mashed potatoes, thick gravy, soft bread, cakes, and pies, stick to teeth and increase plaque and affect its thickness. Plaque, as you know, causes decay and acts as a base for the formation of tartar and gum diseases. The word is: avoid sugar and starches.

How can you recognize plaque? Let's start by describing what it is not. It is not the red or green stains found near the gumline, which are caused by color-producing bacteria. It is not coffee, tea or tobacco stains or tar deposits from tobacco or stains from medication. It is not *materia-alba,* the soft white cheeselike deposit that clings to the plaque on your teeth. It is not food debris. Plaque is made up of mucin, precipitated from stagnant saliva, loose epithelial cells, debris and bacteria. Plaque is generally colorless. However, you can easily identify plaque on your own teeth with the use of disclosing tablets or a disclosing solution (described in detail in Chapter 3).

Since dental plaque acts as a nucleus for the formation of calculus and the initiation of periodontal disease, let's think about the harm plaque can do to gums and to all dental structures. Without everyday oral hygiene, plaque will increase in thickness, complexity and in space. Some people tend to accumulate plaque faster than others under the same hygienic conditions, due probably to a variance in saliva and diet.

TARTAR

If plaque is not removed daily, it will be quick to start an assault on teeth and gums. If it accumulates, it will mineralize or calcify and become hard. The dental profession calls it *calculus* and the layman knows it as *tartar.*

When first deposited, tartar is soft and can still be removed by intensive and prolonged brushing and flossing effort. Eating hard, detergent food products has a modest effect on removal of

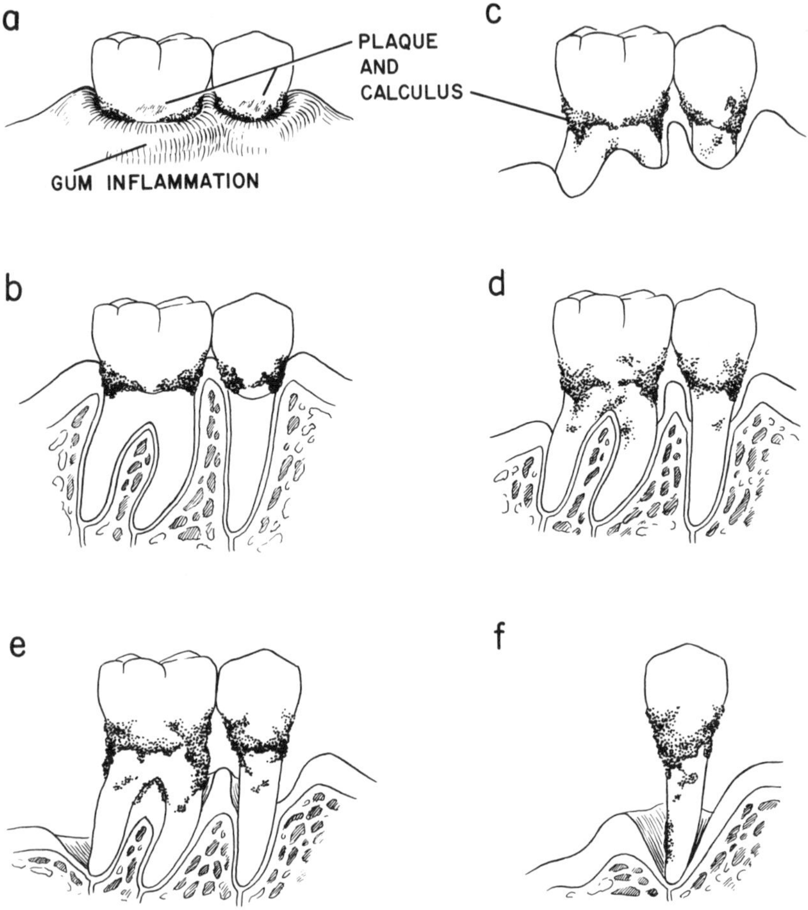

Periodontal disease. (a, b) Plaque and calculus (tartar) deposits accumulate on tooth surface at gumline, causing inflammation. (c, d) Gums recede and inflammation spreads along the roots, with formation of more calculus and pus. (e) Separation of gums along the roots, bone resorption and formation of periodontal pockets. (f) Teeth become loose in their sockets and may fall out.

plaque. However, tartar hardens within a short time and becomes more difficult to remove by brushing. Once calculus deposition has reached the hard stage, it can be removed only by steel instruments. If the deposit is not removed, more tartar will form on top of what is already there and the deposits become larger. The gums become more inflamed and swollen until they almost collapse and separate from the teeth. Deposits of tartar go deeper into the root surfaces and the condition is no longer advanced gingivitis. It is periodontitis, with inflammation spreading along the root of the tooth and bone loss occurring. The tooth becomes progressively looser and is ultimately lost unless professional help is obtained quickly.

If plaque and tartar buildup is discovered when you go to the dentist, either the dentist or the hygienist will scale your teeth. That means the plaque and tartar will be removed from your teeth with the use of small instruments called scalers.

Some individuals are apprehensive; if you are one of those, simply ask for a topical anesthetic. The topical anesthetic is a paste or liquid containing an anesthetic agent which is rubbed around your gums. It also could be a spray of ethyl chloride, which will feel ice cold on your gums for an instant, but that is as it should be. Ethyl chloride acts as a freezing agent to stop pain sensation temporarily.

Scientists around the world have studied the problem and they are in agreement that the more plaque and tartar you accumulate on your teeth, the more chance you have of losing your teeth from periodontitis at any age. Additional causes might be poor diet, especially deficiencies in calcium and vitamin C, certain medical conditions, tooth loss, tooth injuries and heredity. But these factors are secondary. Periodontal disease is the Number One Tooth Killer.

Then comes the question: Why does any sensible person allow his or her teeth and gums to get into such a weakened and hopeless state? The answer could be that they just didn't know any better. And how could they? Periodontitis is a silent, painless killer almost to its last stages. If people are not aware of the symptoms, they have no way of diagnosing the disease.

Any competent dentist will readily recognize early signs of periodontal disease and put a stop to it then and there. Even if he is not a specialist, the dentist can treat your mouth, explain the disease and put you on a program of home care to prevent periodontal disease from recurring. But all hope is lost if you fail to carry out your part by faithfully following the home care program.

Periodontal Treatments

Periodontists are equipped to treat all the gingival diseases discussed in the early part of this chapter. They also treat problems of *occlusal traumatism,* which may be symptomatic of gum disease but do not constitute gum disease. Periodontists can also recontour and reshape areas of bone defects or graft new bone to an area where excessive resorption has taken place. In collaboration with endodontists, they can use sophisticated surgical procedures to perform a *hemisection* (removal of half a tooth) or a *root amputation* (removal of a diseased root) and thereby save many badly diseased teeth. Some of the most common periodontic treatments are discussed in this section.

CURETTAGE OF PERIODONTAL POCKETS

Let's take the case of a *periodontal pocket,* one of the early signs of serious gum trouble. It is exactly what it sounds like, a valleylike opening of gum tissue separated from the side of a tooth's root. Being a pocket, it can and does collect and store many things—mainly plaque, tartar and food.

When the periodontist examines your mouth, the first thing he does is check the depth of the pockets with a periodontal probe; the depth indicates the extent and the severity of the condition. Usually, a neglected mouth will have more than one pocket. Pockets will vary in depth, degree of irritation, amount and severity of bone loss. All these points are vital to the dentist, who will decide on the course of treatment and evaluate its outcome or prognosis.

If disease has progressed, the periodontist may decide to remove the ulcerated layer of soft tissues in the pocket by curettage (a scaling of the tissue) under local anesthetic. Instruments called curettes would be used. Nature and home oral care will do the healing.

When people wait too long to get to the dentist, the periodontal pockets often become so deep and wide that only advanced surgery can save the teeth. If the gingiva has become detached, inflamed and ulcerated, leaving a diseased crevice situated just above the crest of the alveolar bone, the condition is called a *suprabony pocket.* If there is evidence of bone resorption extending below the crest of the alveolar bone, the pocket is called *infrabony.* The pocket is usually large and periodontal fibers have become detached from one or more sides of the root. The diseased area is loaded with tartar, bacteria and infected tissues.

Sometimes the periodontist realizes there is an infection deep in the bone that is supporting a tooth. He may want to scrape, scale, clean or reshape the bone. To get access to the area, he will open the gum tissue in the design of a flap, which exposes the tooth, the root and the bone. After he has operated on the infected bone, the periodontist will bring the flap back and sew it neatly in place.

Gums that have had surgery in this fashion are frequently protected from exposure with a special, cushioned packing made mostly with zinc oxide powder. A piece of foil occasionally is used to cover and protect the packing. This gives comfort to gums which are apt to be quite sensitive. Soft food is recommended. In two or three weeks, a patient returns to the periodontist to have the packing and the sutures removed.

GINGIVECTOMY

Gingivectomy is an operation nobody wants, but a lot of people have in order to save their teeth; the treatment actually is not scary or painful, as some people believe. Briefly, *gingivectomy* involves a cutting away of the gums in order to eliminate periodontal pockets. The operation may be done in one sitting if, for instance, only a few teeth are involved. If your entire mouth is affected, gingivectomy may be performed in several appointments with a different area of the mouth treated in each session. Local anesthetic will be administered before surgery and a packing will be applied to the gums afterward.

A gingivectomy is necessary when all periodontal pockets cannot be scaled, cleaned and curetted completely to wipe out every last vestige of infection. Some pockets are too deep or too irregular to treat effectively; other pockets may be impossible to reach. For example, a pocket hidden in a crater between two teeth could be quite inaccessible. One way to get rid of these pockets is to eliminate them with surgery.

After infected pockets have been successfully removed, the gums may look rather uneven. Since no one wants to show ragged gums when he smiles, the periodontist neatly trims and evens up the gumline. Once this surgery is carried out properly and is completed, a patient should not be troubled again with the disease. But slip up on your oral hygiene and you'll be back to the periodontist. Next time it might be worse.

OSSEOUS RESECTION

Osseous resection is a controversial subject: some dentists like it, others don't. In spite of this controversy, many dentists feel it is worth a try. Keep diseased teeth and diseased bone in your mouth, they say, and you will surely lose your teeth. Reshape and recontour a bone by osseous resection and you're likely to have many teeth for a long time. *Osseous resection* of an infrabony pocket means cutting away the bone to eliminate the diseased pocket. *Bone graft* is occasionally used to repair bone resorption. A word of advice: since most bone problems of this sort are found in pockets between teeth, it pays to work a little harder and longer when cleaning between teeth.

TREATING OCCLUSAL TRAUMATISM

Abnormal hitting or biting of teeth, which results in pathological changes in tissues surrounding the teeth, is called *occlusal traumatism.*

As a rule, lower teeth are touching upper teeth in an ideal, balanced fashion. The occlusal biting force is a healthy force and, when it hits an opposing tooth, the force is equally distributed along the long axis of the teeth to all supporting structures. Occlusal traumatism is encountered in a number of conditions: 1) Several teeth meeting sooner than others when jaws are brought together; 2) An overbite or other types of malocclusion; 3) When teeth are used as abutments for incorrectly designed partial dentures and bridgework; 4) A tooth lost without replacement; 5) A tooth from the opposing jaw forcing itself outward and into the space left by a lost tooth.

Results of these conditions often are occlusal disturbances, trauma, cavities and periodontal disease. Teeth adjacent to empty spaces will drift, tilt, rotate and invite food impaction, cavities, breakdown of gums and periodontal pockets.

Another cause of shifting teeth and occlusal trauma is the action of lip and cheek muscles against the teeth or the force exerted by the tongue. This myofunctional force, only recently recognized and called *myofunctional therapy,* is an upcoming phase in the total treatment of periodontal disease and problems associated with movement and shifting of teeth. Habits such as clenching or clamping teeth can destroy periodontal ligaments and cause bone lesions.

Similarly, *bruxism,* the common habit of grinding the teeth during sleep or even during the day, can wear down the teeth, loosen the teeth, overload the structures, throw the bite out of line, bring on facial pain and cause periodontal disease. A dentist can help a patient with this problem by making a plastic "night guard" to wear over lower teeth at night (and sometimes in the daytime). The protector, similar to the type athletes use, fits over teeth like caps.

Lately, scientists have tried to find a remedy for bruxists. A biofeedback technique, studied at the Facial Pain Research Center at the University of Illinois Medical Center, has been helpful. Persons with the nervous habit have learned to relax their jaws with the aid of therapy and an electronic device which monitors muscle contractions. When the person starts clenching his teeth, the electronic device sounds a beep. This approach seems to be successful, without requiring the use of drugs or any mechanical object in the mouth.

While occlusal traumatism can cause periodontal disease, it also works the other way around—periodontal disease can *cause* occlusal traumatism. Teeth may shift and migrate or they may rise from their sockets and become mobile, resulting in an abnormal, uncomfortable bite. In acute cases, biting or chewing can become so painful that a person may experience great difficulty in eating. The first thing a person so afflicted may think is, "Oh, Lord, let me get rid of these teeth!" Instead, the first thing he *should* think is, "I've got to find a good dentist who can save my teeth!"

In order to effect a cure, every last vestige of periodontal disease must be eradicated and teeth and gums must be absolutely free from plaque, tartar and food debris. The periodontist will study the patient's bite and will grind down the prematurely contacting teeth, then adjust and balance the bite.

For teeth that have shifted, rotated, tilted and are no longer properly aligned, minor surgery or orthodontic correction may be brought into the picture. The periodontist may also employ myofunctional therapy to rid you of damaging lip, cheek or tongue muscle habits.

Many dentists believe in stabilizing loose teeth with wire or splints. Others are opposed to splinting, claiming that it is too difficult for the patient to keep splinted teeth clean.

All evidence today points to dental plaque as the initiator of periodontal disease. Gingivitis, periodontitis and bone loss are more severe in those who have failed to carry out a home oral care program, those who have the greatest accumulation of plaque and tartar at the gum margins.

Periodontal disease can be prevented or controlled. If you have gone through a bout with periodontitis and are healed, never give up visits to your dentist and never let up on your own oral hygiene. Successful periodontal therapy depends on *both* of you.

7 FOUR SPECIALTIES
When you're in deeper trouble

It is comforting to know that advanced dental sciences and technology can diagnose and heal ailments of the mouth, repair damaged tissues and save teeth. Only as a last resort is there a need to sacrifice teeth and make dentures for patients. Four dental specialties are ready to serve you: endodontics, oral pathology, oral surgery and prosthodontics.

The first and most important rule for you to remember is *never* to let a dentist extract teeth to make a bridge or denture. Even saving one tooth is better than saving none. If gums or the entire mouth are in deep trouble, it is your responsibility to control the condition and seek help. Help is as close as a dentist's office.

Endodontics: The Pulp Specialty

An endodontist is a fellow who can save a tooth that might have been pulled 15 years ago. Endodontic treatment has become so successful and is in such demand that many practicing dentists return to dental school for further training.

Primarily, endodontics deals with the diagnosis and treatment of all the conditions affecting the pulp of a tooth. Think of a tooth as having a crown, and a root which anchors the tooth in the jawbone that you cannot see. Under the crown and all the way down along the root is dentin. Inside the dentin is the pulp cavity, containing nerves, connective tissues and blood vessels.

Sometimes the pulp is injured on an athletic field or by a blow to the jaw. Nerves and blood vessels become damaged. A broken or fractured tooth may expose the pulp to harmful bacteria. Bacteria from a very deep cavity or from severe periodontal disease also can infect the pulp and cause the nerve to die. Infection spreads from the pulp to the jawbone and an abscess will develop. To save the tooth from extraction, root canal treatment is necessary.

A good old-fashioned toothache will sound the alarm when pulp is diseased. Toothaches come in two ways: provoked pain and spontaneous pain. The type of toothache will indicate whether the problem is a minor irritation or a more serious inflammation or infection. *Provoked pain,* for example, could occur in a simple gum recession where the neck of a tooth is exposed and is sensitive. Brushing that part of the tooth or even scraping it accidentally will cause a twinge of pain. A recent filling can hurt when contacted by something hot or cold, but the pain will usually go away in one or two months. Both of these provoked pains are minor and nothing much to worry about.

Then there's the kind of provoked pain that makes you jump whenever you eat or drink anything hot or cold, sweet or sour. When provoked pain starts lasting longer—a couple of minutes—it is wise to make an appointment with your dentist. The duration of pain is significant. The longer the pain lasts, the more serious the problem. At this stage, one can begin to suspect a deep cavity, an inflamed nerve or some other flareup in need of immediate attention.

More important is *spontaneous pain.* This pain is either intermittent or constant and it strikes without provocation. For no apparent reason, an individual suddenly feels a sharp pain. The agony may last five minutes or more, vanish and return a few hours later. That's the intermittent variety of spontaneous pain. When the torment becomes deeper and continues for hours, it is constant, severe pain. This could well mean a dying pulp. Emergency care is needed at once. It may be too late to save the nerve, but the tooth can still be saved.

Other toothaches tend to bother us. There's the "long tooth," due to periodontal disease, with pain in the socket. There's referred pain from the nerve. There's intense abscess pain.

Furthermore, many people experience mysterious pain and annoying symptoms in the face that may be difficult to diagnose. Those who have these problems seldom think to question their dentists. Pain and clicking around the ears may be traceable to temporal-mandibular joint dysfunction and is essentially a dental problem. Some persons may be affected with facial pain from trigeminal neuralgia (tic douloureux). If your dentist cannot offer you definitive relief from temporal-mandibular dysfunction, tic douloureux or other types of neuralgia, he or she will refer you to an expert who may help you.

Whenever a toothache strikes, it is imperative to seek help right away. Tell your dentist or endodontist. He will welcome your descriptions of aches and pains, for they will greatly aid him in promptly pinpointing the trouble.

ABSCESSES

When an abscess hits you, you'll know it! The pain is severe and constant, with the side of the face swelling in a few days. This is an emergency. What has happened is that an infection, triggered by tooth decay, has caused the nerve to die. The infection has spread to the bone and an abscess is formed around the tip of the root. This condition is often accompanied by fever.

The endodontist will take over. He must diagnose the origin of the abscess. Is it coming from the devitalized nerve or from the gums? He must control the pain and the infection. If it's from the death of the nerve, he opens the tooth and drains the abscess, and he also lances the gum to drain it. The endodontist may prescribe pain tablets at first, but once drainage begins, pressure is removed and pain subsides. Infection must be controlled or it can get into the blood stream and hence into other parts of the body; therefore, the endodontist may also prescribe antibiotics.

If an abscess is the result of gum disease, the nerve of your tooth is still vital. The dentist will give an injection around the abscess and lance it. He also will scale and clean the involved teeth very carefully.

ROOT CANAL THERAPY AND APICOECTOMY

Almost everybody has heard about it, some of us have had it, but most of us do not know exactly what it's all about. Root canal treatments were performed as far back as the eighteenth century, but usually with little success. Only during the past three decades has the dental profession come up with reliable, scientific techniques and materials that consistently assure a high degree of success in root canal treatment. Presently the success rate of root canal therapy is well over 95 percent.

But isn't it an expensive procedure? Root canal treatment is not cheap, ranging from perhaps $150 to $300. But in the long run, it is much better and cheaper to save the tooth than to have it extracted. The cost of root canal therapy and a necessary filling or crown is less than having the tooth extracted and replacing it with an artificial appliance.

Let's imagine you need root canal therapy. You are experiencing a painful toothache. Although your dentist is competent in treating most teeth needing root canal therapy, he is one of many dentists who choose to refer difficult cases to an endodontist. The endodontist will x-ray the involved tooth. He then will use heat and ice to check the vitality of the nerve. He also will use an electric vitalometer to test the nerve. If the nerve fails to respond, it is nonvital. The sooner the nerve is cleaned out, the better.

And this is how it's done: You may be given a local anesthetic, although some dentists working with very nervous patients may prescribe a sedative or use gas as an anesthetic. Either way, there will be no pain. A rubber dam will be placed over the tooth to prevent saliva contamination and accidental swallowing of small instruments. Also, germicidal solutions used to irrigate the canal will not leak into the mouth. The endodontist will make an access opening through the crown. If it's a front tooth, the opening will be on the lingual surface. If it's a back tooth, the opening will be on the chewing surface. Then the dead nerve will be removed. Using various small instruments called reamers and files, the endodontist proceeds to enlarge and clean out the root canal, readying it for filling.

After cleaning and shaping the canal space until the walls of the canal are as smooth as glass, the endodontist will irrigate the area with germicidal solutions, washing away every last sign of bacteria and infected matter. The canal is dried, medicated and temporarily sealed.

At the next visit, a bacterial culture may be taken, if indicated, to check for the sterility of the canal. When the tooth is comfortable and everything seems fine, the root canal space will be filled with gutta percha, a material resembling rubber. Once the entire canal is sealed, bacteria will not be able to get back into the canal to reinfect it. The abscess will heal completely within 6 months to 2 years.

Since part of the tooth has been cut away, a filling must be placed. Without the nerve and its blood supply, a root-canal-treated tooth needs to be reinforced with a post (a pin or dowel) to prevent fracture and a crown made to protect and prevent the tooth from splitting.

In addition to the regular root canal treatment, occasionally the endodontist may treat a case surgically by doing an apical curettage, or apicoectomy. Briefly, an incision is made in the gum to reach the abscessed area. In an apical curettage, the diseased tissues around the root apex are scraped out. Sometimes the dentist may, for various reasons, perform an

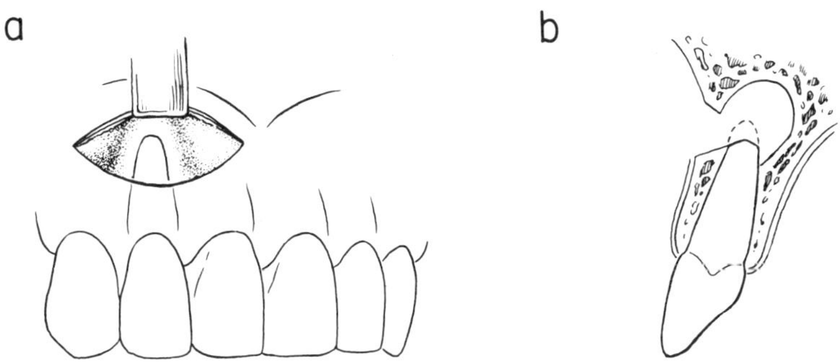

Surgical endodontics. (a) Apical curettage: a tissue flap is made to expose the abscessed area. (b) Apicoectomy: a small portion of the root tip is resected and the infected tissues removed.

apicoectomy by cutting away a small portion of the root tip. This gives better access to the area for the removal of diseased tissues. The gum is then sewed up and stitches will be removed about a week later.

CAUTION: Before having root canal treatment, always ask the dentist what material he will employ to sterilize and fill the root canal. If he plans to use the Sargenti Method or N2 Method, stop him instantly! The Sargenti Method uses a special paste variously designated N2, RC2A, RC2B, etc. The paste contains toxic materials, such as lead, mercury compound and paraformaldehyde. The paraformaldehyde, which resembles embalming fluid, is highly damaging to tissue. If the N2 material leaks out of the root canal, it may travel to other parts of the body and pose a serious lead intoxication threat and other hazards. The U.S. Food and Drug Administration has denied approval of the Sargenti material and is now considering an outright ban. Avoid the dentist who offers a cut-rate price on a root canal filling with potentially toxic hazards. If a dental school is nearby, you can get an excellent root canal treatment at an even lower price.

The average conventional root-canal treatment calls for two to four appointments, depending on the difficulty of the case. When the treatment is completed, you may experience slight discomfort for a few days, but no more than from any other minor operation. *A root-canal-treated tooth is not dead, only the nerve and pulp are gone.* The tooth still gains nutrition through the ligaments that attach the root to the jawbone.

Sometimes your tooth may darken slightly and, if that annoys you, there's a bleaching technique that works pretty well. Or you can have your dentist cover the darkened tooth with a porcelain jacket.

Most root canal failures are due to improper or incomplete sealing of the canal space. A tooth that has been correctly treated and protected will be as strong and as useful as before. The endodontist will want a patient to return every 6 months for x-ray checkups.

Oral Pathology: Treating Mouth Diseases

Do you know much about oral pathology? Few of us do. We become acquainted with this wide-ranging specialty only when

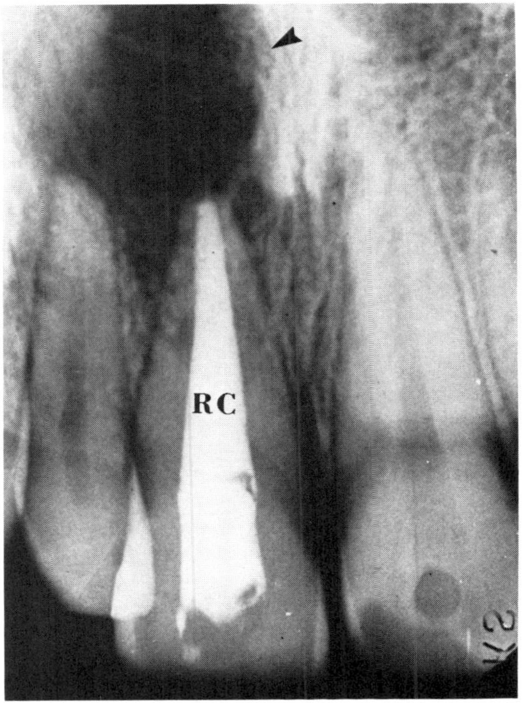

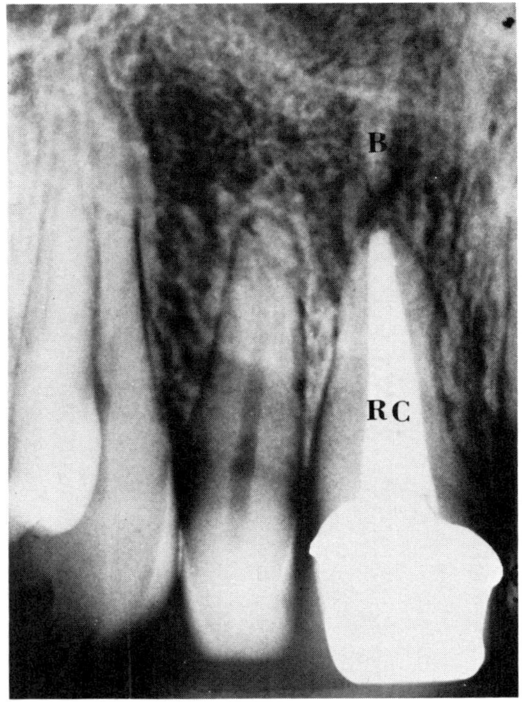

Root canal therapy. (a) X ray of a root-canal-treated tooth showing a large abscess (dark shadow indicated by arrow). (b) X ray of the same tooth one year later: it shows complete healing, with new bone (B) having formed in the previously abscessed area.

a dentist or physician recommends a visit to an oral pathologist. This specialty deals with diseases that are related to the teeth, bones in the jaw, tongue, lips, salivary glands and all other areas inside the mouth.

VIRAL, BACTERIAL AND FUNGUS AFFLICTIONS

Almost everything from plaque and gingivitis to syphilis and cancer come under the oral pathologist's domain. Oral deficiencies and diseases, their diagnosis and treatments, are his field of expertise. Here's a typical case.

While having her teeth checked, a young woman noticed that her dentist was minutely inspecting the inside of her cheeks. Finally, the dentist put down the mouth mirror and casually inquired, "Do you smoke?"

"No, I don't," the woman answered.

"I don't like the appearance of the mucous lining in your mouth," the dentist said. "Do me a favor and see an oral pathologist. It's probably nothing, but it's best to be sure."

Later in the day, the young woman looked into her mouth and saw a bluish-white lacelike network on the inside of her cheeks. She quickly phoned the recommended pathologist. After the oral pathologist had examined her mouth and also taken a biopsy, he told the young woman there was no need for worry. She had *lichen planus*, a minor disturbance sometimes caused by fatigue and nervousness. The young woman slowed her pace and the *lichen planus* subsided.

A mouth can reveal a great many things. Underdeveloped and undercalcified teeth may be a result of lack of vitamins A and D. Painful cracks around the corners of the mouth point to a lack of B vitamins. And without sufficient vitamin C, gum injuries are slow to heal. An oral pathologist may be the first to notice symptoms of scarlet fever, diphtheria, tuberculosis, syphilis or gonorrhea. Scarlet fever shows a fiery red mucous lining and tongue. Grayish membranes appear in the mouth in the case of diphtheria. Lately, gonorrhea cases have greatly outnumbered syphilis; there has been more evidence of gonorrhea in the form of lesions in oral mucous membranes.

A canker sore or *recurrent aphthous ulcer* is a painful ulceration on the moist membranes of the mouth that occurs in school-age children and in adults. Canker sores may appear as single or multiple ulcers, round or oval in shape, with raised, reddened margins. Painful lesions last from 5 to 14 days and heal uneventfully, leaving scars rarely and only in unusually large ulcers. Although the scientific cause is unknown, allergy, inheritance, food intake and socioeconomic status have been suggested as possible causes. A variety of treatments have been recommended. The application of a mild topical anesthetic prior to mealtime will temporarily relieve the pain and make eating less painful. Oral antihistamines and topical application of corticosteroids before meals and at bedtime may be helpful; antibiotic powder from tetracycline capsules may be applied with a moistened cotton applicator and will aid in control of secondary infection. Some doctors suggest that the cause of canker sores is hypochlorhydria, and drinking a glass of water with 10 drops of diluted hydrochloric acid (10%) may give quick relief.

Virus infections of all kinds present still another challenge for the oral pathologist. Probably the most common virus is *herpes simplex,* the one that causes the fever blister or cold sore. Adolescents and young adults seem to get these annoying sores most frequently inside the mouth or on the edge of the lip. The blister may be sore and burning, and you may even feel a little feverish, but it's nothing serious. In 2 to 3 weeks, the blister will be gone. What caused it? A virus. That's all the doctors can tell us. There is no specific treatment, although topical application of corticosteroids may be helpful and antibiotics may be used to control secondary infections.

There are many other viral infections, such as mononucleosis. There is a fungus that can attack the tongue. There are dramatic changes in your gums, lips and tongue if you have a reaction to penicillin. There is *leukoplakia* (meaning white plaque) found in heavy smokers, which is often premalignant. The oral pathologist is truly a Good Samaritan. He sees a condition, recognizes it, treats and heals the condition if it is within his practice. If not, he will direct patients to the specialists who can help.

CANCER

The Dental Health Education Clinic at the University of Pennsylvania School of Dental Medicine has found that more than 30,000 people die yearly from oral cancer, cancer of the larynx, and other head and neck cancers. The main reason malignant tumors are not discovered sooner is because most individuals have not been told how to detect an early growth.

Almost all dental schools have departments of oral pathology, staffed with some of the finest pathologists in the land. If there is any suspicious change in your mouth or throat, your own dentist will direct you to the nearest dental school where a specialist is available to diagnose the condition. Usually, departments of oral pathology in dental schools also offer the public a free self-examination program.

The University of Pennsylvania's self-examination program, a preventive approach, is an admirable example. The technique of self-examination of the oral cavity is simple and may be beneficial. If, during any part of your self-examination, you happen to notice that something looks suspicious—sore spots, lumps, change of color—wait two weeks. If the condition still exists, consult your dentist or physician without delay.

The examination includes eight steps:

1. *Face Symmetry.* Study your face before a mirror. Is there a new lump, bump, swelling, any change of color? Is there a change in a mole or pigment spot? Does your face seem to be proportioned as before?

2. *Lips.* When you press your lips together, do you feel any lumps between your lips? Are there ulcers that haven't healed in the last two weeks? Does the edge of your lip have a normal borderline?

3. *Gums.* Do your gums have any new lumps, bumps, or swellings that do not heal? Ulcers that do not heal? Are there white areas?

4. *Cheeks.* Feel inside your cheeks for any rough areas or lumps or bumps. Do any areas have a white coating?

5. *Tongue.* Are there ulcers with hard borders on the side of your tongue? Are there ulcers or sore spots on the floor of your tongue?

6. *Roof of the Mouth.* Look for lumps, bumps, swellings or sores that do not heal. Notice colored areas that change. Use a mouth mirror and a good lighting source to see well.

7. *Side of the Neck.* Look for lumps that do not go away after two or three weeks.

8. *Center of the Neck.* Your Adam's apple should rise when you swallow. Note any lumps or bumps. Continued hoarseness should be brought to the attention of your doctor.

When detected and treated early enough, most oral cancers are curable. If immediate attention is not obtained, there is a greatly increased chance that cancer will spread into glands and throughout the body.

Oral Surgery: Extractions, Impactions and Injured Teeth

Years ago when you had a tooth problem, out came the tooth. Today, extraction is seldom necessary because modern dentistry no longer considers a problem tooth to be "hopeless." An oral surgeon is busy handling intricate, sophisticated procedures. He is needed to correct such conditions as injury to the

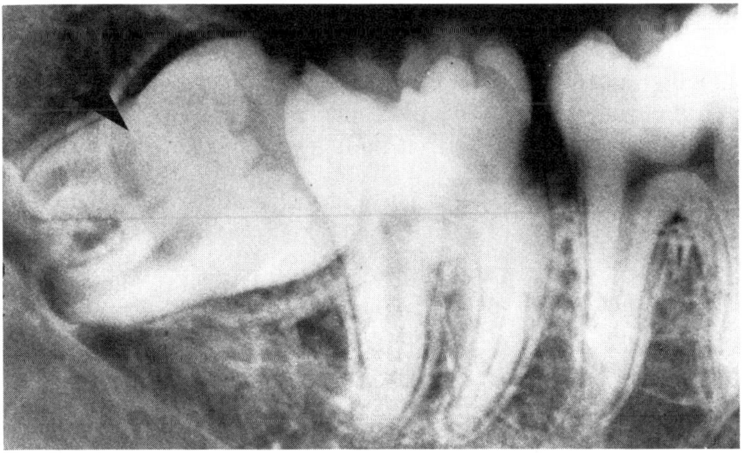

Impacted lower third molar (wisdom tooth) is indicated by the arrow.

teeth and surrounding structures, severe infections and congenital defects. Some surgery can be carried out in his office and, in more complicated cases, surgery will be performed in the hospital.

The oral surgeon is a specialist with extensive training and experience. Like all surgeons, he proceeds in four stages: he cares for you before an operation; he gives you an anesthetic to spare you from pain; he performs the surgery; he gives you postoperative care. He is the man to whom other dentists send their patients when special surgical skills are required. He often collaborates with the endodonist, the oral pathologist and other specialists.

IMPACTED WISDOM TEETH

One of the most frequent surgical procedures is the removal of an impacted wisdom tooth.

Occasionally, the soft tissues surrounding the crown of a partially erupted wisdom tooth may become acutely inflamed and infected. This condition, known as *periconitis,* is very painful and often results in an inability to open the mouth. An extra effort to brush and clean around the third molar, together with frequent rinsing of the mouth with very warm salt water, will reduce the inflammation until you can have the impacted tooth extracted.

The oral surgeon is the man who has the know-how and the specific equipment to do the job. The younger and healthier you are, the sooner you will recover. The surgeon will ask for your medical history so that he is aware of any problems and has an adequate knowledge of your general health. Like other dentists, he wouldn't want to administer the wrong drug or anesthetic.

A local anesthetic may obliterate pain while working around an impacted third molar. Or a general anesthetic—either nitrous oxide gas or an injection of sodium pentothal in a vein—may be used. No matter which anesthetic you get, you will not suffer. The oral surgeon, working with an assistant, will make a flap and remove the impacted tooth. Often a third molar will have three, four or five curved roots. The surgeon may section the tooth in several pieces to get it out.

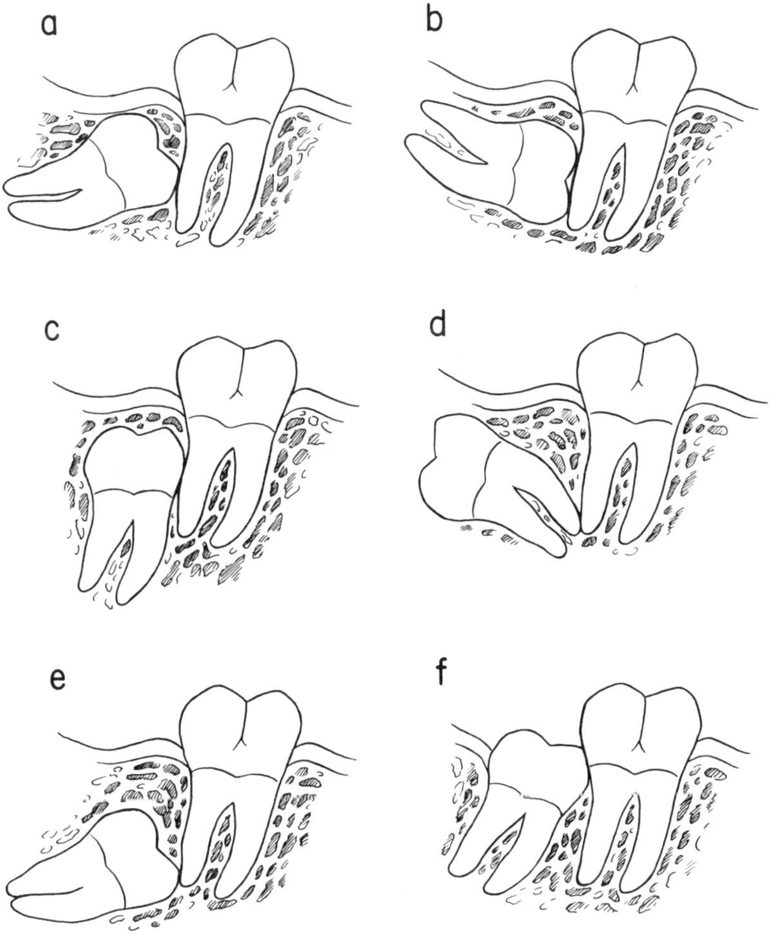

Examples of impaction. (a) Mesioangular. (b) Horizontal. (c) Vertical. (d) Distoangular. (e) Low level. (f) High level.

He then proceeds to carefully clean out any tooth chips, bone fragments or foreign matter. The wound is irrigated and closed with sutures. Bleeding usually is minimal. You may have a little pain and some swelling of your jaw for a few days.

TUMORS, CYSTS AND MALIGNANCIES

There are many instances when an oral pathologist has diagnosed infected cysts, tumors and other disorders in a person's mouth and then turned the case over to the oral surgeon. Oral pathologist and oral surgeon, combining their talents, are able to treat and cure pathological conditions which, left unattended, could become extremely serious.

Prosthodontics: Replacing Missing Teeth

Many dentists will make replacement teeth for their patients, but if your mouth is difficult to fit with a bridge or dentures, you may need the expertise of a specialist, a prosthodontist. A prosthesis is the artificial tooth, bridge or denture. Prosthodontists also construct appliances to help plastic surgeons replace eyes, noses and other parts of the face.

Suppose you've lost a tooth. You don't like the way your mouth looks and you know very well that if you don't replace that lost tooth soon, other teeth are going to move, tip and turn, and the dental arch will collapse. It's something like removing one brick from an arch of a building. Wisely, you go to a dentist or prosthodontist, who may advise a bridge. There are several types of dental bridges: the fixed bridge, the cantilever bridge and the removable bridge (partial denture).

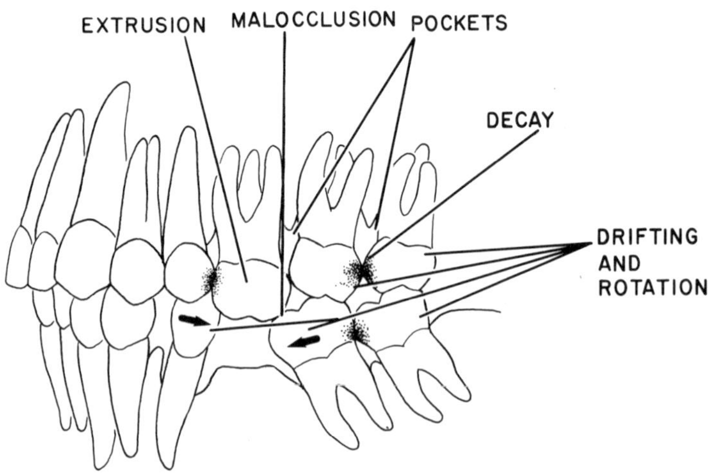

Possible results of the failure to replace a missing tooth with a prosthetic appliance.

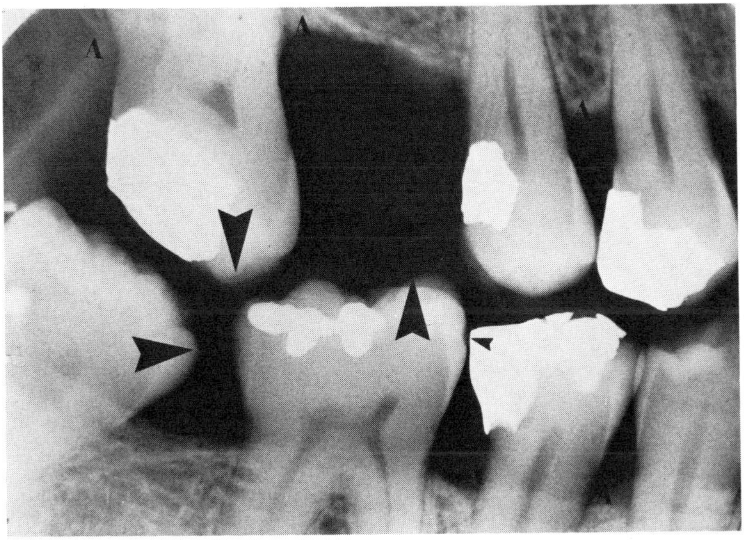

X ray of the mouth of a 35-year-old person showing what happens when a missing tooth is not replaced with a bridge or partial denture. Large arrows indicate drifting teeth which create food impaction areas where decay starts. Periodontal disease with bone destruction can be observed at areas marked A.

FIXED AND CANTILEVER BRIDGES

The best prosthesis to replace one lost tooth is the *fixed bridge*. This is how it's done. The teeth on either side of a missing tooth will act as pillars and are called abutments. These abutments will be worked on first. The prosthodontist will prepare abutments to hold the bridge. The bridge, if desired, can be constructed with no metal showing. The specialist will fit the bridge onto the abutments and let the patient examine it with a mirror. *If for any reason, a patient is not satisfied, this is the time to speak up.* If the appearance of the new bridge is satisfactory, the dentist will cement it in for keeps.

The cantilever bridge is a one-abutment bridge. The crown is fitted on the abutment tooth and the pontic is soldered to the crown or the bridge frame is made in a one-piece casting. The pontic—the part of the bridge that spans the space—replaces the missing tooth and sits snugly against a healthy tooth on the other side. Cantilever bridges are not as stable or as good as fixed bridges.

Your new fixed bridge may feel awkward because the tongue has had time to "spread" a little bit into the area where the tooth was missing. It will take some time for the tongue to regain its original shape, but the feeling of bigness and the sense of interference by the bridge will disappear.

You may experience a feeling of pressure on the teeth to which the bridge is anchored, making these teeth sore temporarily. It is also not unusual for the anchor teeth to become sensitive to hot or cold liquids, cold air, or even brushing, particularly near the gumline. In some cases, the dentist can apply various desensitizing drugs to these areas. Sensitivity will last for some time, until nature builds up an insulating area within the anchor teeth.

No matter how well a bridge is made, food debris is likely to collect around the edges. You should be aware that, in time, gums and bone may shrink, causing space to develop under the bridge. It is important to spend several minutes cleaning around and under the bridge. If you cannot get floss between the gum and the tooth, food debris cannot get in either.

With a medium-soft, small-headed toothbrush, scrub the tops and sides of the bridge, moving the brush in all directions to clean all parts of the teeth. You should also brush the gums, because this massaging increases circulation in the gums and bone and helps keep these tissues in a healthier condition.

Dental aids are available for threading dental floss between bridge and gum to effectively keep the area clean. These floss threaders are needlelike, flexible nylon loops. Take a piece of dental floss or tape about 20 inches long and insert it into the floss threader. Push the straight end of the threader carefully through the space between the artificial tooth and an anchor tooth. When the straight end passes through the space and toward the tongue side, reach inside the mouth and pull the threader and the floss through, then slide the loop off the floss.

Wind one end of the floss around the index finger of one hand, grasp and lock the other end of the floss in the other hand by winding it around the middle, third and small fingers. Insert only the two fingers or finger and thumb in the mouth to manipulate the floss. Maintain a short span of floss between the fingers as you guide it along. Move the floss gently between the gum tissue and the artificial tooth or teeth to clean the underside of the bridge.

Then move the floss against the side of one of the abutment teeth. Press the floss against the tooth and, with a sweeping motion, move it up and down to clean the side of the tooth. Then guide the floss between the gum tissue and the artificial tooth to the side of the other abutment tooth and repeat the procedure. You might want to ask your dentist to demonstrate the proper technique and to watch while you do the job effectively.

While you have the floss handy, you might as well floss all your teeth. The oral irrigating unit, which furnishes jets of water under pressure, is a useful appliance to flush food debris from between teeth and gums around bridgework.

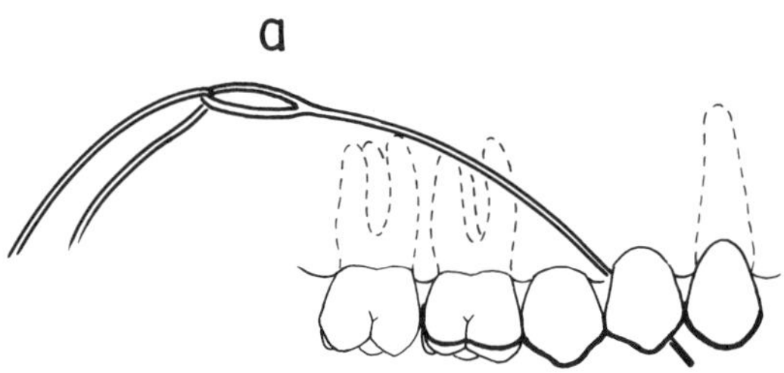

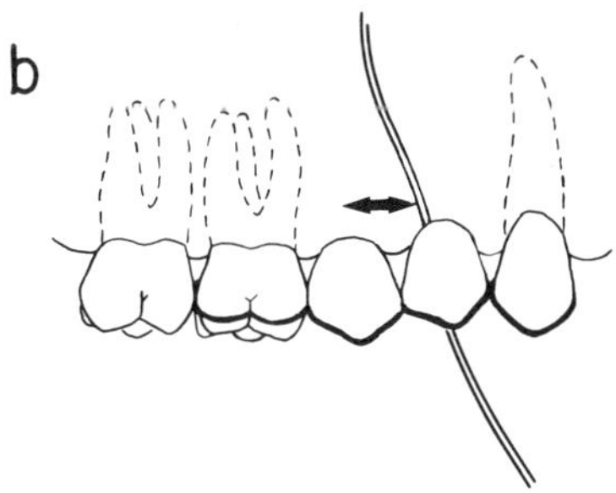

Flossing a fixed bridge. (a) Using a floss threader and about 18 inches of floss, pull 4 or 5 inches of floss through loop of threader. Pass threader through space under the bridge. (b) Work floss between the pontic and the gum. (c) Floss the adjoining surfaces of artificial and abutment teeth.

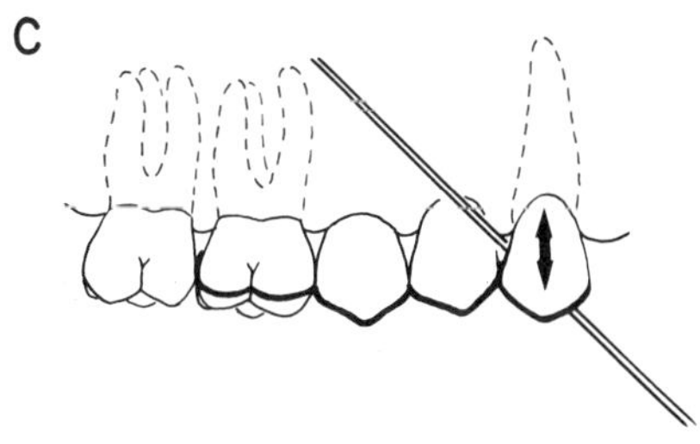

A word of caution about a fixed bridge for a child or a young adult: in young people, the dental pulp is quite large and, since the abutment tooth must be reduced considerably, cutting may reach close to the nerve. The tooth may become sensitive to heat and cold and the nerve may be affected. It is better for a young person to use a temporary removable bridge. As a person gets older, the dental nerve tends to shrink and there's little or no risk of nerve damage when the fixed bridge is constructed.

PARTIAL DENTURES

Because a fixed bridge is the most expensive type, some people will decide on a less costly partial denture or removable bridge. The partial denture is an artificial appliance with clasps to fit onto the existing teeth. Many people prefer partial dentures without visible clasps. They are fitted into the abutment teeth by a precision attachment device and are more costly. Partial dentures are usually more extensive and replace several missing teeth. If an individual has lost all back teeth, a fixed bridge cannot be made since there is no posterior abutment onto which the bridge can be attached. We will discuss the possibility of implants for fixed bridgework in Chapter 10; routinely, however, the loss of back teeth calls for a partial denture.

Without back teeth on one or both sides of the jaw, it's difficult to chew efficiently. Also, when there are no upper back teeth to bite against the lower back teeth, the lower back teeth gradually will work out of their sockets and end up hitting the upper gums, making it impossible to fit a denture. If a partial denture is not made, the remaining teeth will carry a greater work load and break down sooner, leading to premature tooth loss.

Partial dentures may be made entirely in acrylic or with a cast-metal frame. The frame may be of gold or a nonprecious metal. Gold partials cost more, but are more flexible and easier to adjust.

There is a great difference between well-made, intelligently designed partial dentures and poorly designed dentures. A poorly designed partial will cause food impaction, tooth decay and gum disease, and will rock the abutment teeth loose. As the areas where the clasps fit onto the teeth are more susceptible to decay, it is important to spend a little extra time thoroughly cleaning the abutment teeth of a partial denture.

A partial denture used for the first time seems bulky and annoying, but people get used to it quite readily. Chewing becomes easy. A denture should be removed and washed thoroughly with soap or toothpaste and toothbrush after every meal. Preferably, it should be placed in a glass of water overnight to give the mouth a rest. The best-fitting partial denture will become loose with repeated use and should be tightened by your dentist every few months.

FULL DENTURES

If you have read and heeded this book in time, you will never need full dentures. If, unfortunately, you have lost all your teeth, look for the best dentist or prosthodontist available and have him fit you with comfortable, natural-looking dentures. Good dentures require skill, patience and time to construct. A well-made set can be finished in no less than six to eight appointments.

Avoid dentists who advertise dentures in 24 hours. These dental plates usually are ill-fitting and seldom satisfactory. Wise consumers do not go to denturists—dental lab technicians who illegally make cheap dentures without taking into consideration the patient's medical and dental problems.

A good prosthodontist will take time to evaluate your general and oral health and the shape of your face. He will check your mouth for inflammation, tumors, impacted teeth or retained root tips. He will then have a clear picture of the type of teeth to be used in the denture you—and you alone—will require. The dentist will work closely with laboratory technicians, who will follow his instructions. When the dentures are finished, the dentist will want you to return to his office if you have the slightest difficulty.

For most people, it's a shock to lose all their teeth, but one can gradually adjust to the change. At first, when the new dentures are inserted in your mouth, you probably will notice that there is considerable facial change. You will look as though you have "too much teeth." However, after a few weeks, the muscles will readjust themselves. The upper lip with lengthen, covering the teeth, so that less of the upper front teeth will show. Your mouth will shape and mold itself so that a softer facial appearance will be noted. You may find that the dentures feel particularly bulky and that the tongue has been restricted in its action. There may be a tendency to gag, due to the fact that the tongue is forced into the throat. There is nothing to worry about, since the tongue—which has enlarged considerably after the removal of the teeth—will shrink down to normal size again in due time. If you experience gagging, just close the teeth together and breathe very slowly, trying to occupy your mind with some pleasant thought. In a short time the average denture wearer will not be troubled by gagging sensations.

Gagging may also be due to an excessive amount of saliva of a ropy nature. Rinsing the mouth with a saltwater solution, using about half a teaspoon of salt in a glass of warm water, will control gagging in most cases. The dentures should be replaced in the mouth and not removed until further rinsing of the mouth is required.

You may find your speech affected to some degree because of the thickness of the denture base. Difficulty in speaking clearly can be overcome by reading aloud to yourself, carefully pronouncing the syllables of each word, and placing special emphasis on their enunciation.

Eating. Some patients experience difficulty in learning how to eat with new dentures because they expect them to be similar to their natural teeth. It is best not to eat foods that are hard to chew until the dentures have been adjusted by the dentist so they feel comfortable in your mouth and no sore spots exist. While you are waiting for an appointment, pain from sore spots may be relieved by applying Campho-Phenique to the areas with a Q-Tip and by rinsing the mouth with warm saltwater a few times a day. Be sure to wear your dentures at least 12 hours before the appointment. If you do not wear the dentures, the sore spots will not be recorded in the mouth. It will be impossible for the dentist to determine and correct the source of difficulty.

You will have to cut food into relatively small particles and learn to take smaller bites. It will be necessary for you to learn to chew entirely on your back teeth, rather than attempt to use your front teeth to chew food. It is best to start with hamburger, fish or ground foods which do not require a tremendous amount of chewing.

In due time, you will master the trick of eating apples, pears or corn-on-the-cob. When eating corn-on-the-cob, you reverse the rotation of the cob and turn the cob against the upper front teeth, actually scraping the corn off the cob. The back portion of the tongue, pushing against the back of the upper denture, will hold the denture securely in place. Very little pressure is placed on the food with lower anterior teeth. In biting into an apple or a pear, the same technique is used. Most of the force is directed against the upper front teeth, while the tongue holds the denture up at the back.

Cleaning. It's best to wear your dentures every day, all day long. Continuous wear will fill out your cheeks and lips and give you a natural, younger appearance. Dentures may be kept in the mouth at night if they are comfortable. Otherwise, leave them out at night, put them in water and let the mouth rest. A few drops of household bleach in a glass of water will reduce denture stains and make dentures smell sweet and fresh.

Proper hygiene is absolutely essential for maintaining healthy gums in denture wearers. Twice a day, remove the dentures and massage the gum tissue with a soft brush or a washcloth moistened in water. This massage will stimulate the circulation and maintain the health of gums.

While you are massaging your gums, the dentures can be placed in a solution made by adding a half-teaspoon of household bleach to a large glass of water. The dentures are then removed and scrubbed with ordinary bath soap or toothpaste or powder. Dentures may break if they are accidentally dropped into the washbasin. It is a good idea to place a washcloth in the bottom of the basin and fill the basin with several inches of water to protect the dentures in case they slip out of your hand. This treatment of the dentures, carried out several times each week, will ensure clean, odorless dentures and will greatly facilitate the removal of food stains, plaque and tartar which can form on artificial teeth, as well as real ones.

Relining. When a considerable amount of mouth recontouring has taken place, it is very desirable to have the denture rebased to fill the space between denture and jawbone. Rebasing gives a better fit, maintains healthy gums, discourages the formation of flabby tissues and lessens the rate of bone resorption. People with tender gums can turn to dentures that are relined with a soft acrylic base for more comfort.

Repairs. Do-it-yourself repair of dentures can be dangerous because some of the products used have seriously harmed many people. Also, broken sections can be difficult to reassemble correctly and one may end up with an ill-fitting denture. It is best to have the dentist repair dentures correctly and recheck the bite, because breakage of teeth or breakage of the entire denture is often due to change in the occlusal relations of the teeth.

Adhesives. If a denture becomes slightly loose, denture adhesives may provide temporary help. However, long-term use of denture adhesives on very loose dentures is undesirable. Loose dentures promote excessive growth of flabby gum tissues and bone loss, making it difficult to fit a new denture. It's better to have dentures properly rebased as soon as they begin to fit poorly.

The life of a set of dentures varies considerably with the individual; they may last from 1 to 15 or 20 years. Denture material may discolor or become brittle. The mouth may undergo changes, dependent upon the general health of the individual. The jawbone may shrink, resulting in loose dentures and a considerable change in facial appearance. On the average, the usefulness of a set of dentures is from 3 to 5 years.

After 3 or 4 years, denture teeth wear down and, with gum shrinkage, more wrinkles appear. If this happens, it is time for a new set. Poorly constructed dentures can cause injury to the gums and may contribute to the development of oral cancer. Wearers of loose-fitting dental plates due to extreme bone loss can now anticipate tighter-fitting implant dentures.

8 PEDODONTICS
Children's dentistry

The modern-day pedodontist has shed the traditional white coat and the stuffy, clinical manner that went with it. His reception room is painted in cheerful colors. Furniture is scaled for the little folks. There's a rocking horse in one corner, stuffed toys in another, piles of comic books and games to play. Music from the stereo is nursery rhymes or rock-and-roll. Dr. Jones greets his patients, aged 1 to 15, with a big smile. The kids call him "Doc". The profession calls him a pedodontist.

Primary Objectives

What exactly is pedodontics? It's dentistry for children only. The objective is to care for very young patients and especially to teach them and their parents oral hygiene and preventive dentistry. Pedodontists believe that early prevention is vastly more efficient than treating tooth and gum problems later in life. A child's first visit to a dentist is usually at the age of 2 to $2^1/_2$ years, although some dentists are suggesting that age one is none too early. It is a fact that 1-year-olds already have a few teeth and plaque can accumulate on those teeth. Another fact is that 50 percent of 2-year-olds have one or more decayed teeth.

A parent should definitely be concerned about a young child's teeth, because primary teeth lay the groundwork for permanent teeth to follow. That's why a parent should bring a child to a pedodontist while he's young. Early instruction in home care tops the list of priorities. As soon as possible, teach your child home oral care. Although, of course, you will be doing most of the brushing and flossing at this stage, make it a fun venture, a part of acting like the grownups.

There's another reason for getting your child to the pedodontist. Your child, like thousands of others, may have the habit of *thumb* or *finger sucking*. A most natural instinct, to be sure. But if it's carried on much after the age of 4, it may become harmful to the teeth that are coming in and it may also affect the shape of the growing jawbone. *Tongue thrusting* is another undesirable habit. Thrusting the tongue through the teeth can push them out of alignment and cause the teeth to become crooked.

Some parents are still unaware of "nursing bottle mouth." If a parent continues to put a tot to sleep with a bottle full of sugary liquids (formula or soft drink), he is contributing to early cavities. The longer a child cries for the sweetened bottle and the more often the bottle is thrust into the mouth, the more damage will be done. The poor kid may end up with teeth so badly decayed they will need to be extracted.

Mixed Dentition: Primary and Permanent Teeth

Let's talk about those primary teeth. They start coming in when an infant is approximately 6 months old and they are all in at about the age of 2 or 2½ years. Don't ever think of deciduous teeth as unimportant. They are very important. You know that they prepare a foundation for permanent teeth and there are other reasons for taking excellent care of them.

A child will be unable to chew his food thoroughly if his teeth become decayed, infected or extracted.

Cavity-ridden teeth or lost teeth make a child unattractive to

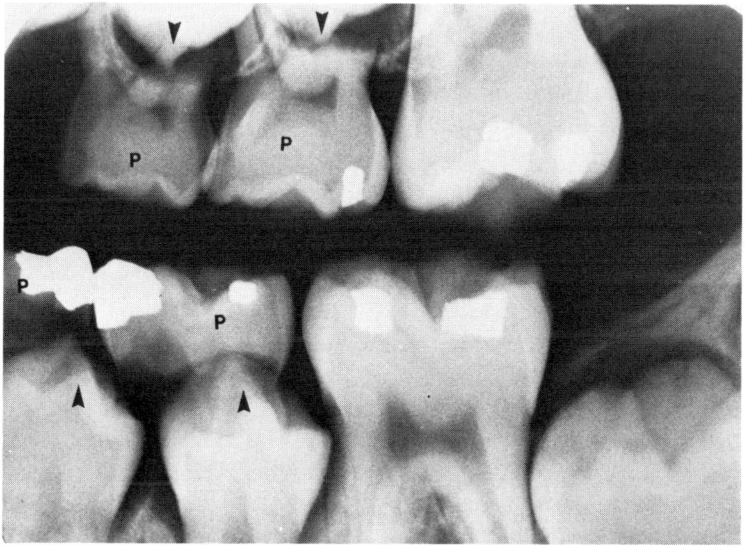

Bitewing x ray showing mixed dentition in a 10-year-old child. *Ps* indicate primary teeth with root resorption caused by permanent teeth pressing against them. Arrows indicate erupting permanent teeth.

other children. Infected or lost teeth may also cause deformities in facial development and expression.

If a primary tooth is lost too early, other primary teeth will drift into the space. That will throw the permanent teeth out of alignment and they are likely to come in irregularly, due to lack of room. Also, a child needs baby teeth in order to speak properly.

While all primary teeth are in by the age of $2\frac{1}{2}$ at the latest, it is the sequence rather than time of eruption that is of major significance. Variations in the pattern frequently are the causes of poor bites.

From the age of about 6 to 12, there will undoubtedly be some primary and some permanent teeth in a child's mouth at the same time. This situation is called *mixed dentition.* As a child grows, the face grows, too. It grows downward and forward. Girls' faces grow faster than boys'. Usually all permanent teeth are in, except for wisdom teeth, by the age of 13.

Fluoride application to help build up resistance to cavities starts at about the age of 3 and continues to the age of 15. If drinking water has the proper fluoride content, this topical fluoride treatment may not be essential. In spite of fluoride, however, cavities do appear. And early.

Parental Roles in Early Hygiene

Many studies on the toothbrushing habits of children have shown that preschool-age children brush their teeth too briefly—less than 20 seconds. They have not developed the skills to handle the brush so that they can perform efficient toothbrushing. Likewise, the performance of children under 7 years was found to be more brief and haphazard than that of older children.

It was also reported that parents brush a child's teeth significantly better than the child himself. Most dentists agree that for primary dentition—children under 5 years—the horizontal or scrub technique seems to remove plaque better than the vertical (up and down) technique. For the mixed dentition of older children, the vertical technique (from gums to chewing surface) is recommended.

When brushing a child's teeth, have him stand in front of you, leaning back with his head resting on your left arm. Use the fingers of your left hand to retract the lips and cheek. The right hand is free to brush all the surfaces of both anterior and posterior teeth.

When brushing the upper teeth, ask the child to tip his head back to give you adequate vision. Again, the fingers of the left hand are used to retract the lips and cheek. You can look directly into the mouth while brushing the teeth with your right hand. If the child is very small or you are very tall, you can sit on a low stool. In this position, you can brush the child's teeth with more comfort.

As you recall, the 6-year molar, the last tooth immediately behind the primary teeth, is the first permanent molar. It is, unfortunately, often mistaken for a deciduous tooth and negligently cleaned. According to statistics, the first permanent molars are most susceptible to decay and are often lost early in life. The extra minute you spend to thoroughly brush the back molars of children 6 years or older will prolong the life of these most important teeth.

After you have brushed and flossed your child's teeth, encourage your child to also brush. It is a good idea to ask your dentist or the plaque control therapist to show you and your child the proper toothbrushing and flossing technique. You can also learn how to identify plaque that has not been removed, then how to remove it.

The Youngster and His Dentist

Most dentists prefer not to have a parent accompany the child in the patient room. Dentists like to start off a friendly, trusting relationship with a young patient to eliminate fear and to put the youngster on an adult level. In this way, he is able to have the child think positively about dental care.

As with adults, x rays are necessary to check for any hidden disorders. If there's only a tiny cavity to be filled, the procedure can be finished in half an hour or less. Parents are often overly concerned about the child's experience in having the first filling. The child, on the other hand, actually will have been a good, cooperative patient.

Should a primary tooth ever be extracted? A primary tooth acts as nature's space maintainer, holding down the parking place for the permanent tooth to come. That primary tooth should never be extracted if there is any chance at all of saving it through careful treatment. However, if the tooth is so decayed or infected that the condition could be harmful to the child's health, the pedodontist likely would extract it.

Leaving an empty area after extraction would start other teeth drifting—it's nature's effort to close up the gap. To halt drifting, the pedodontist will insert a space maintainer where the permanent tooth will eventually erupt. A space maintainer may be removable, fixed or semifixed.

At about the age of 6 a child is apt to lose his front teeth and, at the same time, his first permanent teeth—the first molars—erupt. These molars are called the 6-year molars and are the sixth back from the center of the mouth. They do not replace primary molars. They are on their own for life. They are the largest and most important teeth of all, for they are the keystones of the dental arches. But for a child to reach back to them and clean them properly is not easy, which is unfortunate. Of all teeth, *the first molars are the most susceptible to cavities.* They bear little grooves on their chewing surfaces that readily collect and hold destructive plaque. For this reason, first molars are the teeth that decay the most and are often extracted early in life.

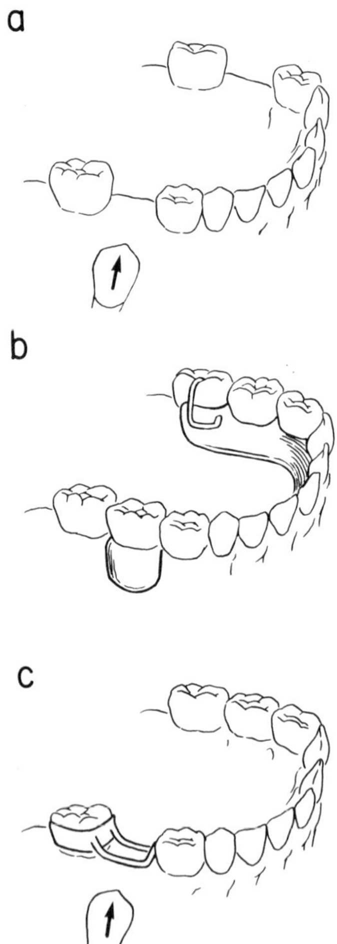

Space maintainers. (a) A primary tooth was extracted, leaving an empty space. Arrows show bud of an erupting permanent tooth. (b) A removable space maintainer preserves the space where the permanent tooth will eventually erupt. (c) Fixed space maintainer band and loop type.

Children should have regular checkups with their pedodontists. Shortly after the 6-year molars erupt, the pedodontist may recommend coating the chewing surfaces with a pit and fissure sealant. The sooner, the better. Reliable statistics tell us that at the age of 7, approximately 25 percent of lower first permanent molars and 12 percent of upper first molars have cavities.

When all permanent teeth, except wisdom teeth, have erupted, 13-year-olds begin to face a critical period. At the time when home dental care is needed most, teenagers are neglecting their teeth. Their diets consist mostly of junk food and far too much sugar. Inevitably, tooth decay follows and permanent teeth are on their way to ruin. Fluoride may help, but is not the entire answer. The longer the neglect, the larger the cavities. Furthermore, there may be problems of periodontal disease, a need of orthodontic treatment or perhaps even minor surgery. If a youngster ignores the need for dental care, he'll be very sorry by the time he's 17 or 18 and wants to have attractive-looking teeth.

Young people may think of periodontal disease as something that only older folks have. Not true. It can strike anybody at any age. If the disease is caught early enough, the pedodontist can heal it. If the condition becomes severe, a youngster will require the services of a periodontist to save his teeth.

There is sometimes a problem with teeth not following the normal pattern of eruption or alignment. Here pedodontics and orthodontics overlap. Frequently, a pedodontist will handle cases of preventive orthodontics and interceptive orthodontics. *Preventive orthodontics* is aimed at warding off any harmful changes in the natural course of development. An experienced dentist, by the use of selective serial extractions of primary teeth, can often circumvent future orthodontic treatment and save many thousands of dollars for the parents. If a youngster has very deep cavities between teeth, resulting in loss of tooth structure, teeth would collapse against each other, then drift, with resultant changes in the dental arch. The pedodontist must clean out the cavities and build up the teeth to maintain a healthy arch.

When a youngster's bite develops incorrectly, *interceptive orthodontics* may be required. A space maintainer is used to reposition a tooth that has drifted or tipped and is preventing another tooth from coming in straight. Too, the pedodontist is alert to continued childish habits, such as thumbsucking, that might cause teeth to protrude or other disorders. The pedodontist usually has a friendly chat with his young patient, explaining the harm. If the young patient doesn't drop the habit or outgrow it, there are remedies to help him overcome the problem.

Teenagers, particularly those who are athletically inclined, far too often come home with a fractured or broken tooth after a football or hockey game. The kid is in pain and it is best to rush him to his dentist or pedodontist. If the fracture is not extensive and there is still vitality in the pulp, the tooth may be restored with a crown. If the pulp dies, the tooth may still be saved by endodontic treatment.

If a tooth has been completely knocked out, luckily, it can sometimes be reimplanted. Youngster or adult, it's good to know how to save such a tooth. Do not take time to wash the tooth; just pick it up, put it back in the socket, if possible, or under your tongue, and hold it there until you can get to a dentist on the double. The sooner that tooth is replaced, the better the chance of successful reimplantation. There have been numerous cases where a tooth has been replaced in its socket immediately and has reattached itself and lasted for many years. Delay in replantation will increase chance of failure due to root resorption.

Incidentally, any child or teenager involved in contact sports would be wise to wear a mouth protector.

All children and teenagers should see their dentists twice a year, just as adults do—or should. Good healthy teeth are essential for good healthy living. Preservation of primary teeth is vital for the completion of root formation of permanent teeth. As soon as permanent teeth are in, they should be watched and cared for as if they were precious, irreplaceable gems—in a sense, they are!

9 ORTHODONTICS
Not for children only

The correction of irregularly aligned teeth is called orthodontics. This specialty is concerned with diagnosis, causes, prevention and realignment of teeth that have grown crooked, tilted, far apart, or simply do not fit each other. Orthodontics also means correcting jaws that are underslung or protruding, and jaws that do not work together properly.

Orthodontia is not just cosmetic dentistry: correctly aligned teeth are less prone to cavities and have the best chance of remaining healthy for a lifetime. Periodontal disease is much less likely to develop and the entire supportive system is healthier.

Malocclusion: Inherited and Acquired

Occlusion means the proper fitting together of the lower and upper teeth when they are in normal contact. *Malocclusion* is any abnormal relation of teeth in one arch with those of the opposite arch when the jaws are closed. If not corrected, malocclusion can lead to deformities of face and jaws and may have an adverse psychological effect on a young person for life.

How important is it to have youngsters' teeth straightened? As children grow up, they begin to hate their buck teeth or crooked teeth, stop smiling and sometimes wind up with an emotional problem as bad as the malocclusion itself. Because chewing can be difficult, a youngster may swallow without chewing or may select only soft foods. Then nutrition is inadequate and digestion of food incomplete. Sometimes with malocclusion, a youngster's jaw joints and muscles will be strained, causing discomfort.

If that isn't enough incentive to have a child's teeth straightened, consider the difficulty in oral hygiene. How can a person brush teeth that overlap and are overcrowded? Bacteria and plaque get in where a brush cannot. Dental cavities and periodontal disease follow quickly and destructively.

Statistics indicate that 50 percent of children in all age groups need some form of orthodontic care. Malocclusion is first noticeable when permanent teeth begin to erupt. The condition is recognized as crowded teeth or teeth spaced far apart; protruding upper or lower teeth; front teeth that don't meet when back teeth meet, or vice-versa. Although parents and teachers occasionally spot these abnormalities, hopefully the child has been visiting the pedodontist regularly. A pedodontist will certainly recommend orthodontic treatment when indicated.

Some people need orthodontia and some do not. Those who don't are just plain lucky. The others can blame their malocclusion primarily on heredity. Each parent has different traits: you may inherit one trait from one parent, another from the other parent or perhaps a forgotten one from a grandparent. It's unlikely that your mouth will be exactly like that of your mother or father. With your father's large jaw and your mother's small teeth, you're apt to have unattractive spaces. It's not too unusual to have one tooth a different size than its mate on the other side. All this is *inherited malocclusion.*

Acquired malocclusion is brought on by neglect, certain diseases, a deficient diet, injurious habits or prenatal influences, such as German measles. Habits are the most prevalent. You should understand that living bone is somewhat like plastic. It can be molded by pressure. That means a child's jawbone can be unnaturally distorted by sucking and biting habits, as well as always sleeping with one jaw on an arm or resting the jaw on a hand for long periods.

Habits are formed right after birth and that perhaps is the time to keep the good habits and banish the bad ones. A certain amount of thumb and finger sucking is normal for an infant, but as the infant becomes a child, the habit becomes abnormal and harmful. Any continued pressure on the teeth or the bones of a child's face may cause irreversible damage. One or both jaws may develop improperly and teeth are apt to be displaced. In any of these cases, the pedodontist and orthodontist are there to intercept and correct the condition before it develops too far.

Orthodontic Correction and Appliances

First of all, the family dentist or the pedodontist will recognize the need for orthodontic correction. Teeth normally come together somewhat like meshed gears. When teeth fail to occlude correctly, chewing is inadequate and a string of problems follow. A continued faulty bite causes undue stress on certain teeth. The bite causes damage to gums, to supporting structures and to the jaw joints. If the family dentist and the pedodontist cannot help the young patient, he is sent to the orthodontist.

Age is not a factor, because every case is entirely individual. A 5-year-old child who has prematurely lost a baby tooth might be a candidate for the orthodontist's chair. Most youngsters get into orthodontics when they're 12 to 14. However, some people show up for correction as late as in their 30s and 40s.

With a young child or teenager, a parent or both parents are asked to be present for the first visit to the orthodontist's office. There is always a need for the understanding and cooperation of child, parents and orthodontist as the treatment goes along and it's wise to start off with that in mind. During the first couple of visits, the orthodontist will discuss his plan of treatment, the fees, the length of time involved, his role in the correction, the child's and parents' roles. Unless the child is quite young, most orthodontists prefer that a parent does not tag along at each appointment. Children seem to be more at ease, too. Parents, however, are welcome to occasionally accompany the child to observe what's going on and how the treatment is progressing.

After the orthodontist has examined and x-rayed the child's teeth and has studied the dental and medical history, he will make a plaster cast of the patient's teeth, gums and jaws. He will also take measurements of the patient's face and take photographs. The "before and after" photos will later show how the treatment has improved the patient's appearance.

Fundamentally, there are three broad classes of malocclusion. Two of the classes refer to overbites and the third to underbites. With an overbite, the front upper incisor and canine teeth project over the lower teeth and the lower jaw recedes. With the underbite, the front lower incisor and canine teeth project over the uppers and create an undershot or lantern jaw.

Correction is accomplished by moving the teeth into their normal positions. The principle of tooth movement is based on pressure, either intermittent or constant. There are various methods to move the teeth into satisfactory position. A particular malocclusion may respond better to one kind of mechanical device than to another. Orthodontic appliances may be made of stainless steel or acrylic. Stainless steel may be coated with plastic to render it less conspicuous. Rubber elastics, chin straps and headgear are often used along with orthodontic appliances.

Once the orthodontist has made his diagnosis and planned his treatment, he will select the proper orthodontic appliance for the particular case. He then will fit the patient with the fixed appliance, usually banding all permanent teeth. He can manipulate certain brackets on the appliance to gradually move an individual tooth in any direction required. Youngsters will feel some small discomfort in the beginning, but it soon passes. There is never any real pain. Orthodontic treatment may last two years or more.

During this time, the youngster should try extra hard to keep the teeth very clean. While the bands cover and can protect some areas of the teeth, they also catch and hold food. Parents are asked to cooperate by seeing that a child maintains extra good oral hygiene and to discourage eating foods such as sticky, sugary candy. Occasionally, a band may become loose and have to be recemented. Loose bands, not recemented, allow food to collect and cause decay. Youngsters with this condition should see the orthodontist as soon as possible and, in the meantime, thorough cleaning, including conscientious brushing, flossing and flushing, is imperative. Regular examinations by the dentist or pedodontist, of course, should be continued simultaneously, as it is most important to catch the beginning of any cavity. After the bands are removed, a retentive device is generally worn to stabilize the teeth in their new positions. The device is known as a retainer. These retainers are removable and after a while the patient wears them only at night and, finally, not at all.

When it's all over, the rewards are many. Teeth are functioning as they should. Appearance has been improved. The entire mouth—teeth, gums, supporting structures—is in a much healthier state than before. It becomes a lot easier for a youngster to brush and floss and home dental care can be carried out much more effectively. In almost all cases, proper orthodontic treatment succeeds in bettering a youngster physically and emotionally.

Orthodontia for Adults: Special Considerations

Today, many adults are seeking the orthodontic treatment their parents could not afford to provide years ago. Others are having their teeth straightened to gain a more comfortable bite, to be able to clean teeth more satisfactorily, to have less cavities and periodontal problems and thereby preserve their teeth. Also, dental insurance has made orthodontic work less costly for the patient. Whatever their reasons, adults now account for 20 percent of the average orthodontist's practice.

But there are problems. Jaws and teeth have almost stopped growing and orthodontic movement is usually slower. There can be pain. There are limits to how much teeth can be moved: too great a force or too much speed of movement can cause damage to the surrounding tissues, root resorption and devital-

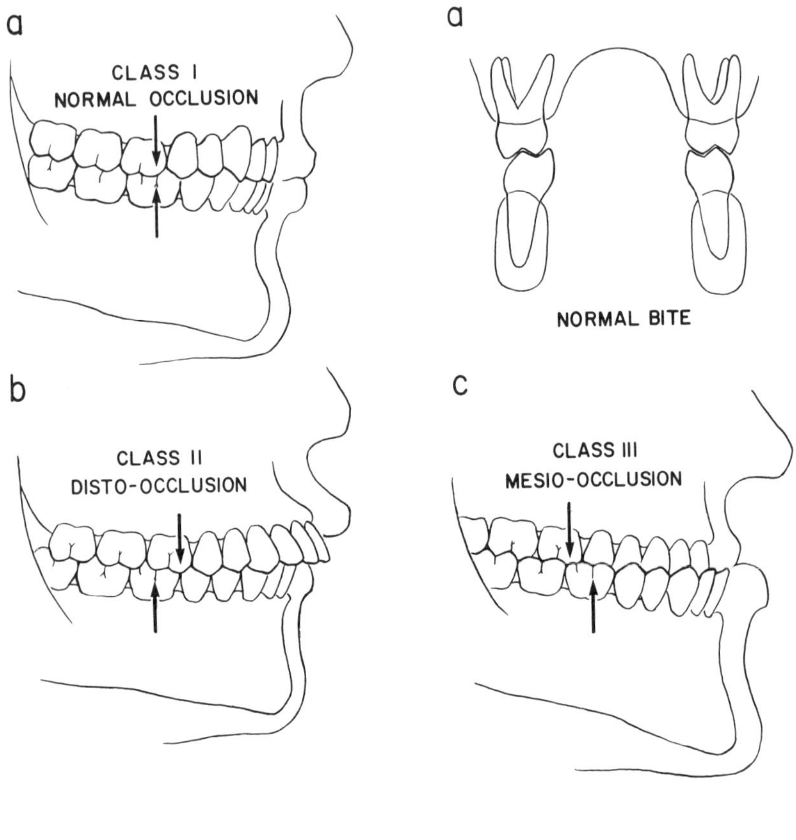

ized teeth. There is also a chance of relapse. Children are luckier. Their teeth and jaws are still growing and the moving of teeth can be coordinated with their growth patterns.

Then is it worth the trouble, the discomfort and the cost ($2000 or more) for adults to have their teeth straightened? Yes, according to many orthodontists. And many adults have discovered their straightened teeth are far healthier, less likely to get cavities and periodontal disease than crooked, poorly positioned teeth. They have also discovered that time and money spent on fillings, root canal therapy, etc., would, over the years, add up to a lot more than an orthodontist's fee. Lastly, your own straight teeth have the best chance of hanging in there for a lifetime.

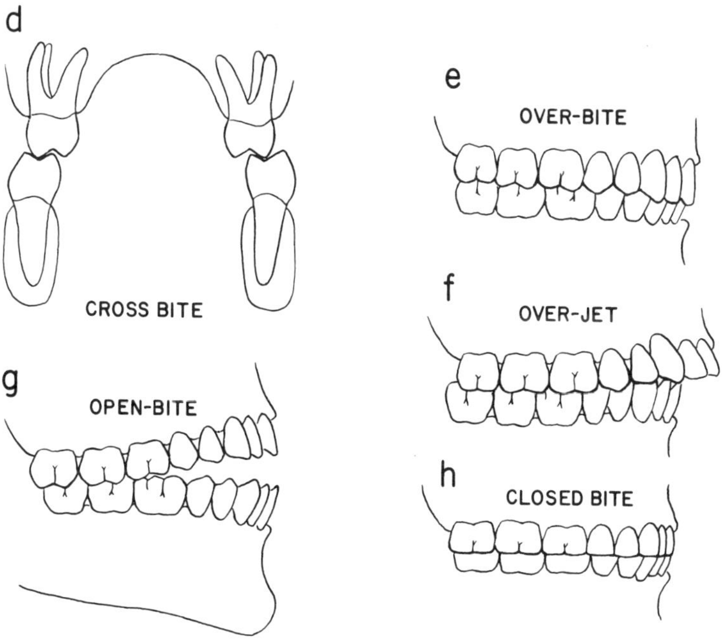

Occlusion and malocclusion. (a) Profile and cutaway views show the normal occlusal relationship of the teeth. (b) Distoocclusion, protruding upper teeth. (c) Mesioocclusion, jutting lower teeth. (d) Crossbite. (e) Overbite. (f) Overjet. (g) Open bite. (h) Closed bite.

10 SPACE-AGE DENTISTRY
The future is now

Within the last two decades, dentistry has passed from the era of extraction, bridgework, dentures and reparative therapy into the era of prevention of disease, cosmetic dentistry, tooth implants and other remarkable advances. These innovations have been brought about by dedicated dental teachers and researchers, with particular contributions from a group of little-known specialists in the field of dental public health.

The Public Health Specialist

Public health, one of the eight specialties in dentistry, deals primarily with studies of the causes, extent and treatment of dental diseases. For example, the thousands of studies on fluoridated water brought the public one of the most significant and valuable rewards ever. Dental public health deals also with education and treatment of the public in different communities. Specialists may have dental degrees, medical degrees, or doctorates in highly specialized fields. Unlike practicing dentists in the other seven specialties, this specialist is concerned not with a small number of patients, but rather with large groups of the population.

The public health official often may be found in a community of low-income families where dental disease has long been neglected. The specialist goes to work educating the community and locating dentists nearby to volunteer their time. He outlines ways in which the community may finance an office building and dental equipment from its budget.

A specialist may head a large dental clinic funded by the city or county. He then assumes the dual role of superintendent and teacher. He may lecture, publish informative booklets on oral care, prepare audio-visual aids, such as slides and motion pictures—all in an effort to effectively educate the public.

The research specialist may be deeply involved in searching for a certain cure, testing a new material, evaluating new dental equipment. Whatever the project, the specialist is the pathfinder, the discoverer of great breakthroughs. Research in our space age has produced tremendous advances in dentistry and has given the public the advantages of painless drills, wonderful filling materials and tooth-saving discoveries.

All these achievements could not be realized without financial aid from the federal government, state and city governments, individuals and foundations.

Dental Schools and Clinics

In recent years, there has been a steady increase in dental schools. Presently, some sixty American dental schools graduate almost 6,000 new dentists yearly. New schools are modern in every way and older schools are constantly updating physical facilities, equipment, materials, teaching concepts and curriculum. In step with today's thinking, many schools have added courses on preventive dentistry and community dentistry. Some have even created an entire Department of Preventive Dentistry, representing a significant segment of the curriculum. Although a need will always exist for excellent restorative dentistry, the emphasis on repairs is a thing of the past. *The new breed of dental graduates firmly believe in and advocate preventive dentistry above all else.*

Dental schools have public clinics. Advanced students work on patients under close faculty supervision. In this way, individuals in the community can take advantage of good and inexpensive dental care. The cost of treatment in clinics is considerably less than the average fee in a private office. Furthermore, a dental school's clinic can offer the most up-to-date techniques and a variety of services, including oral examination and x rays, all types of fillings, root canal treatment, bridgework, removable appliances, oral surgery, dentistry for children, orthodontic treatment, periodontic treatment, facial reconstruction, oral cancer detection and emergency treatment.

One of the most dramatic services offered by a dental school is the mobile dental clinic. The project, started only a few years ago, is the concept of Dr. Marvin M. Stark of the University of California, San Francisco. Dr. Stark took an old house trailer, converted it into a dental clinic on wheels and, with dental students, traveled back roads to give dental aid to children of migrant workers.

Today, with large sums of money donated by corporations and concerned individuals, modern buses are outfitted with the latest dental equipment and staffed by volunteer dental students and dental instructors from the University of Michigan and the University of Southern California, as well as from UCSF.

In another innovative program, a new mobile dental clinic and staff journey to a foreign country, donate their services and eliminate needless pain in children. Before the staff leaves, the mobile clinic is presented to the country. Israel, Greece and Yugoslavia have benefited.

Trends in Private Practice

PLAQUE CONTROL CENTERS

Plaque control centers are becoming increasingly prevalent. New dentists are so geared to preventive dentistry that, when they open their offices, they frequently reserve one room as a patient education and plaque control center. The room is likely to be small with a row of wash basins, a large wall mirror, excellent lighting, teeth cleaning materials, teaching aids, movies and microscopes. The dentist, an assistant or a hygienist acting as a control therapist gives patients a thorough demonstration and practice course on plaque control. It's a course patients find definitely worth the time, effort and minimal fee.

FILLING MATERIALS

Appealing to both dentist and patient is the emergence of extraordinary filling materials. These new materials have resulted in the simplification of a number of restorative procedures. The result is easier, quicker, more efficient repairs. Also, they conserve tooth structure, cause less pain, are more economical and look more natural.

One of the most popular fillings is an adhesive composite material. No longer does the dentist need to perform tedious cutting and make retentions in cases of erosion or small cavities. All he has to do is clean out the cavity and etch the tooth enamel with acid. The material and its bonding agent are applied to the etched, roughened surface, then shaped to the contour of the tooth. It is exposed to ultraviolet light, which will harden the material. This filling has color stability and demonstrates excellent resistance to wear from brushing. Many severely fractured front teeth have been repaired successfully with the adhesive material and without the need of undercuts or retaining pins. Composite materials easily match tooth shades. They do not discolor and they stand stress well. Although the pit-and-fissure sealants are still in an experimental stage, they appear to be durable and effective. Unique varieties of plastic and porcelain materials also are working well.

If an artificial tooth in a plastic or porcelain bridge is chipped or fractured, it can be repaired in the mouth without having to remake the entire bridge. A dentist works with the plastic or porcelain material as though it were putty, contouring the restoration to his satisfaction.

CHARACTERIZED DENTURES

For those seeking the most realistic appearance in dentures, *characterized dentures* are available. These are not average dental plates where every tooth is straight, even and pearly white. Characterized dentures are made to look natural, showing normal wear. An indentation here, a stain there, a slightly crooked tooth, a gold filling. The base of the denture can be tinted and stippled to have the appearance of real gums.

Business is brisk in these customized teeth, made either of porcelain or plastic. Porcelain teeth look better than plastic, because they reflect more light. Porcelain wears better, but the newer, stronger plastic teeth are gaining in popularity. With teeth greatly improved and enhanced, individuals find dentures much more acceptable, even if it means paying many times the average price. In spite of added cost, characterized dentures make up 35 percent of all dentures.

Invisible Orthodontics

In the old days of orthodontia, bands made of stainless steel were very conspicuous. Today, the profession is switching to the barely noticeable plastic materials. Youngsters are much happier. Adults, who would never be caught wearing unsightly metal bands, have succumbed to visiting the orthodontist. Science has found a way to coat orthodontic materials with tooth-colored plastic. Plastic brackets can be cemented directly and securely to tooth surfaces with new bonding agents. Even space maintainers can be almost invisible.

Cosmetic Dentistry

Discolored or stained teeth can be restored to their original color. Discoloration may be due to the death of the nerve, the use of certain antibiotics (tetracycline discoloration) or overfluoridated water. In some cultures, prolonged use of native foods and beverages have been known to darken teeth. Bleaching techniques employing concentrated oxidizing agents, such as hydrogen peroxide and other chemicals, have been success-

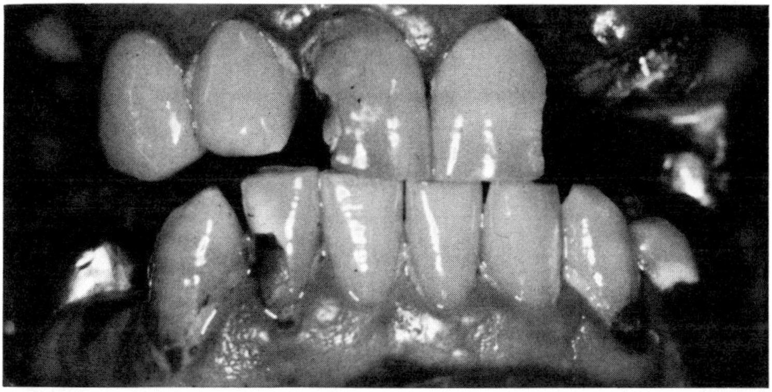

Before and after pictures demonstrate what modern dentistry can do. Reconstruction was accomplished without extracting the badly broken down teeth. Even the fractured tooth (top right) was saved by performing root canal therapy and building a stump over the root. Teeth were covered with porcelain fused to gold crowns.

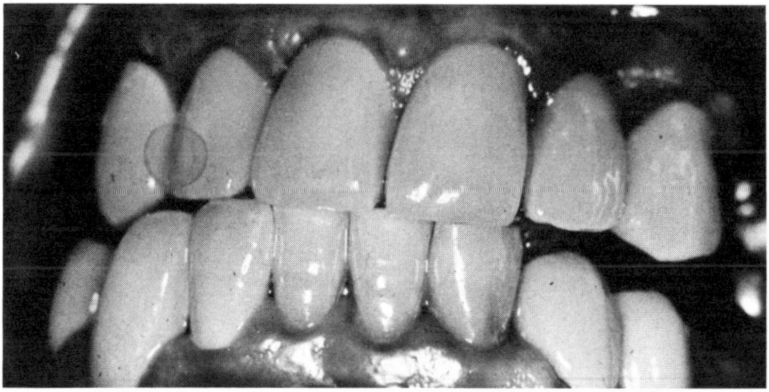

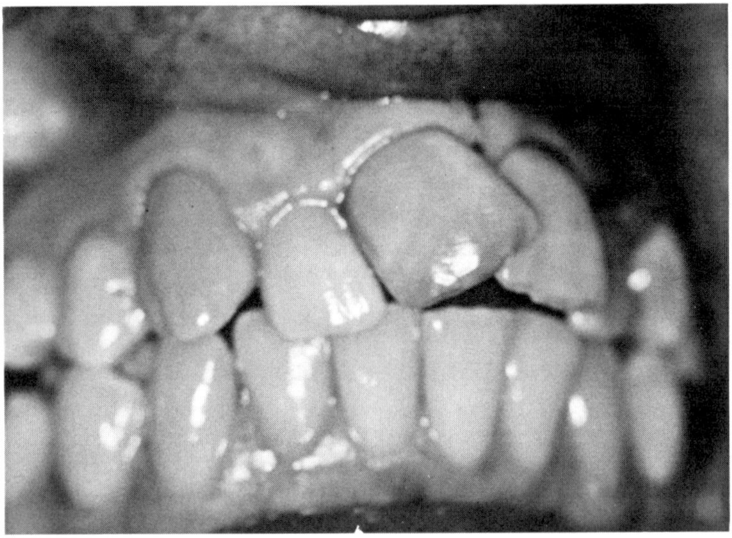

A extremely crooked tooth in an adult mouth (top) can be quickly and permanently "straightened" and repositioned correctly with the use of porcelain fused to gold or porcelain veneer crowns. (Bottom) after cosmetic dentistry.

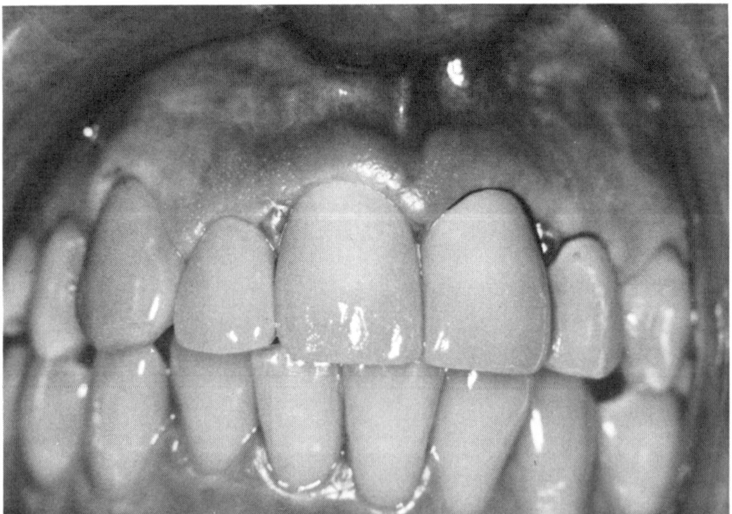

ful in most cases. Bleaching is much more economical and conservative than capping teeth.

Dentistry is cosmetically oriented these days. The public is turning away from gold crowns and bridges. "Take them out! Gold ages me!" patients tell their dentists. Everybody seems to want beautiful teeth, and they can have them. More unique than ordinary porcelain caps and bridges is cosmetic reconstruction and rearrangement of teeth. If front teeth are crooked or overlapped, or if one tooth is spaced too far from another, the dentist can align them perfectly. A simple case might be the existence of considerable space between two teeth. Each tooth is made wider by adding adhesive material to the sides of the teeth until they contact. Or the teeth can be capped to eliminate the gap.

More skill and time is required to reconstruct a long tooth or crooked teeth. A long tooth cannot be shortened without cutting too close to the pulp. Therefore, in some cases of cosmetic reconstruction, root canal treatment is applied. After the nerve is removed and the canal filled, the dentist can safely cut off the end of the long tooth so that it matches the length of the others.

The most challenging of all cosmetic reshaping of natural teeth is the transformation of a crooked tooth into a straight one. A very crooked tooth in an older person can seldom be satisfactorily straightened by orthodontic means. As the crown of the tooth must be reduced considerably to make it look straight, root canal treatment is needed and the tooth must be reinforced with a dowel. A cap is sculptured to fit in a normal position over the prepared tooth. While the unseen root will remain at its original angle, the visible cap will be straight.

Office Equipment

Only with the steady flow of scientific discoveries and inventions has modern dentistry been able to produce so many wonders. Dental offices have a space-age atmosphere. Walk into a modern patient room and it will be empty except for the colorful dental chair, which slides on rails and can automatically raise or lower a patient's head or feet. Lights appear mysteriously from the ceiling and the dentist's instruments are hidden in the walls, ready to slide out when needed. Drills make a silent appearance from hidden panels and disappear when their job is done. The whole idea is to do away with the tacky, old-fashioned office where the first things a patient saw were ominous drills and a tray full of menacing instruments.

Today's drill runs at 500,000 rpm without vibration. It can cut a tooth like butter and completely prepare a small cavity in two minutes. Some drills have fiber-optic lights attached, providing the dentist intensified light for excellent vision. Ultrasonic equipment is being used. There is an ultrasonic scaler that scales teeth and an ultrasonic electrosurgical kit which enables a dentist to cut a gum without causing pain or bleeding. Straw-colored latex tubing has been developed to cover the wire often used to stabilize loose teeth. The tubing not only masks the wire, it protects the mouth from irritation. Dentists, assistants and hygienists are changing their appearance, with white coats and uniforms gradually being replaced by personalized attire. The direction is toward modernization in every aspect of the office.

Oral Implants

Implantology, or implant dentistry, is probably the most significant forward step in dental practice. When all means of good prosthetic dentistry and periodontal treatment have failed to provide stable appliances for a patient, the prosthodontist can use implant prosthesis.

Basically, oral implantology is a two-stage procedure. The first stage is inserting the implant abutments either on the surface of the jawbone *(subperiosteal implant)* or in the bone *(endosseous implant).* The implant is a specially designed blade or a stud made of a special alloy (titanium, palladium, etc.) or of vitreous carbon that is inserted into healthy bone. Part of the implant protrudes over the gums and looks like a tooth that has been prepared to receive a cap.

The second stage is fabricating and placing the denture (or bridge) over the studs or abutments. This is accomplished by having corresponding snaps fastened to the base of the denture.

The appliance snaps over the protruding studs and gives the denture excellent support and a stability not previously experienced by the patient.

At this writing, oral implantology is in its early stage of development. Further studies and careful analysis of a patient's medical and dental history, as well as long term followups of cases, must be carried out. In selected cases, however, implant prosthesis has proved to be an extremely happy experience for the patients.

Another type of implant, using *endodontic stabilizers,* is done through the root canal to enhance the retention and prolong the life of a loose tooth. The endodontist drills a hole through the root canal and extends the drilling into the jawbone. He then cements a rigid implant rod in the canal, giving additional length to the root and stabilization to the loose tooth. A root canal treated with endodontic stabilizers makes an excellent abutment for a bridge or a partial denture.

Overdentures

There is a new way to make dentures which vastly improves the retention of dental plates and has become a boon to denture wearers. Hopeless teeth are no longer extracted. Instead, root canal treatment is performed, then the teeth are cut down to the level of the gumline. The roots of the teeth remain imbedded in the jawbones and the presence of these roots prevents the alveolar bone from shrinking. This preserves the ridges and gives good retention and support for the dentures.

Another method is to cement metal studs on top of the embedded roots. The studs protrude perhaps 1/4 inch. Corresponding snaps are fastened to the denture. All the individual needs to do is to snap the denture onto the studs and there are no more worries about dentures slipping.

Tooth Replantation

Replantation is the replacement of a tooth in its own socket. There are several types of replantation. A tooth knocked out in an accident and replaced in its own socket is *nonintentional replantation. Intentional replantation* is planned extraction, endodontic treatment and replacement of the tooth in its own socket. The purpose is to save the tooth. If the procedure is carried out rapidly and correctly, the replanted tooth can last many years.

There are two other remarkable replants, *autogenous* and *heterogeneous.* If a young person, for instance, has a completely broken-down first molar, the oral surgeon will extract it, then proceed to extract the young person's healthy wisdom tooth. He replants the wisdom tooth in the socket left empty by the molar. This technique is *autogenous replantation.*

In a *heterogeneous replant,* a donor is required. If an individual loses a tooth, a young brother, sister, or friend can donate a wisdom tooth for replantation. Due to widespread interest, tooth banks are being set up in many regions. Tooth replantation has met with varying degrees of success; at this writing, it should be considered in the experimental stage.

Hypnotism and Acupuncture

Anesthetics have come a long way since cocaine was the best available pain killer. Modern anesthetics are fast-acting, effective and available, yet some people tend to look into the past for ancient means the world has half forgotten. Hypnotism and acupuncture are indeed used today and with a certain amount of success. Hypnosis is known to work when dentist and patient are both tuned into mind expansion. However, in fast-paced dentistry, time consumed in putting a patient under hypnosis is not profitable. Nor is it very popular.

Acupuncture anesthesia has created considerably more enthusiasm. Can it be the dental anesthesia to surpass all others? Its proponents claim it is safe, simple and economical. Nothing more is needed than a few needles placed in the correct areas of the body. American dentists who have witnessed tooth extractions under acupuncture anesthesia in the People's Republic of China have reported there was little or no evidence of pain. Nevertheless, dentists concluded that acupuncture is no better than our fast-acting anesthesia, except for patients with heart trouble or some allergic conditions. The ADA further cautioned that the use of acupuncture is premature and continued laboratory and clinical investigations are needed.

Experimental Concepts

We cannot ignore some of the fascinating experimental materials and theories that may be accepted any day. A device known as the ultrasonograph detects dental cavities by means of sound waves at 15 megacycles a minute. Such a machine could prove to be more efficient than x rays.

Scientists are testing antiseptic mouthwashes that may prevent plaque and decay from forming. Another promising experiment concerns vaccine to prevent tooth decay. Tests have demonstrated positive results. Also, root canals can be filled in less than a minute by injecting plastic materials into the prepared canal. These plastic materials show excellent tolerance by body tissues, with no interference with bone healing and repair.

There are controversial sugar substitutes in chewing gums, the latest being Xylitol, which has been found to reduce tooth decay. This substance is many times sweeter than sugar and is on the Food and Drug Administration generally regarded as safe (GRAS) list. However, Xylitol has been reported to cause cancer in mice by the National Institute of Dental Research. As a result, all human tests to see whether Xylitol reduces tooth decay have been suspended.

As a parting word of advice, remember that dental disease is more easily prevented than cured and that you and only you are in control of your mouth. Neglect of your mouth is expensive in terms of health, happiness and money. A good preventive oral hygiene program on a sustained basis rewards you by keeping your mouth healthy and your smile attractive.

The greatest changes in the future of dentistry seem to revolve around the practice of preventive dentistry. We can anticipate a time in this century, when there will be no cavities, no need for repairs. All teeth and gums will be healthy, strong and beautiful.

11 DOCTOR, TELL ME . . .
101 questions and answers

Is it true that an unborn baby already has teeth?

Yes. At four or five months gestation, an unborn child has twenty tooth buds, ten in each jaw, beneath the gums.

Why do I feel something like mist in my mouth when I yawn?

There's a salivary gland under your tongue and two more glands under your ears. When you open your mouth wide, glands are squeezed and out comes a spray of saliva.

If I accidentally bite my tongue and it bleeds, what should I do?

Rinse with warm saltwater every hour. The bleeding usually stops in a few minutes. If it's a nasty bite, put a little Campho-Phenique on the spot two or three times a day.

Is there a new method of charting teeth?

Lately, American dentistry is numbering teeth. Counting from the upper right wisdom tooth to the upper left wisdom tooth are numbers 1 to 16. The lower left wisdom tooth is 17, the lower right wisdom tooth is number 32 (see Chapter 1).

Do we inherit our teeth from our parents?

Yes, inherited genes affect teeth. Fluoride in drinking water, diet and oral hygiene habits make a great difference in the teeth you inherited, though.

Why do some people have very white teeth and others have darker teeth?

Individuals have different pigmentation in their teeth, as well as in their skin.

Why do teeth turn yellow as we grow older?

The nerve gets smaller, the dentin gets thicker, the enamel gets thinner and the yellow dentin shows through. There are also stains that accumulate from foods and beverages.

Can I have an impacted tooth I don't know about?

Yes, although it will always show up on x rays. Otherwise, you are seldom aware of it until it causes trouble.

At what age do baby teeth become loose and start to fall out?

At about 7 or 8 years of age.

Why have some of my teeth moved back to their original positions after orthodontic treatment?

If teeth have been moved too quickly, new bone in the sockets may not have had enough time to form. Therefore, it is extremely important not to give up the retainer too soon.

Is it all right to hold things like pencils, carpentry nails or safety pins between your teeth?

Not a very good idea. You'll tend to chip your teeth. This is called "wear and damage due to habits."

I do a lot of sewing and I bite off thread with my teeth. Any harm in this?

It is known that seamstresses wear down the biting edges of their front teeth by constantly biting thread.

When I eat, I frequently bite the inside of my cheeks. Why?

Biting your cheeks sometimes occurs when you eat too rapidly. But usually this happens when you have a new crown, dentures or bridgework. It takes time to adjust to something new in your mouth.

Is chewing on only one side of your mouth harmful?

It is likely. Teeth on the preferred side are subject to more stress and may break down sooner. Check with your dentist.

What is the purpose of brushing your teeth?

Toothbrushing promotes good oral hygiene, helps prevent the gums and teeth from becoming diseased and gives your mouth a healthy, clean appearance.

Why do some people have more saliva than others?

You have more saliva when you are young. As you grow older, the salivary glands are not so active. Some diet elements and drugs can influence saliva flow.

Is there sugar in toothpastes?

Most toothpastes contain sweetening agents, such as sorbitol and/or glycerin, but not sugar.

Why are my teeth sensitive to heat and cold sometimes, but not always?

After cleaning and scaling or eating certain fruits, teeth may become sensitive for a short while. A new restoration may cause the same reaction, but should disappear in time.

If the edges of my front teeth are jagged, should I have them smoothed off by grinding?

Yes. If you don't, the teeth will chip and become even more jagged.

Is it permissible to chew ice cubes?

It's not a very good habit, since it's possible to crack or chip your teeth. Try sucking instead of cracking on ice and, if you must chew, do it very gently.

What dental products should I take on a trip abroad?

Antibiotics to which you are not allergic and some strong pain tablets in case of infection, abscess or any emergency; also, several toothbrushes, dental floss, toothpaste, salt.

Is vomiting harmful to my teeth?

Yes. It brings strong acid into the mouth which can cause the teeth to decay. It's best to rinse your mouth as soon as possible.

How does fluoridation help prevent cavities?

Fluoride in the water supply can be incorporated into the enamel of a young child's forming teeth. This makes the enamel slightly harder and more resistant to dental decay.

What is a "dead" tooth?

It is an imprecise term, really meaning the *nerve* in the tooth is dead.

Why do teeth decay more than other parts of the body?

The mouth can almost be considered a garbage pail. It contains bacteria, thriving on the sugar and starch which we constantly provide. No other part of the body offers such a fertile field.

Who gets more cavities—men or women?

Cavities affect both sexes equally. The difference depends on the care you take of your mouth. Women seem to have somewhat fewer, probably because they are more religious about seeing a dentist regularly.

Can I tell when I have a cavity?

Not always. Sometimes an early cavity doesn't hurt and an x ray is necessary.

Why do sweet foods hurt when they contact a cavity?

Because of the difference in osmotic pressure between the sweet and the tooth structure. When the sweet contacts the decayed tooth, the flow of osmotic action causes pain.

Are artificial sweeteners harmful to teeth?

In general, no. But there is need for further research in this area.

Can an adult benefit from fluoride?

Yes, but not to the extent of children's teeth, since the enamel has already been formed by the time you reach adulthood.

Does vitamin C help your gums?

Absolutely. It helps heal tissues of the gums and plays an important role in the formation of all membranes.

Is it all right to chew vitamin C tablets?

It is better to swallow them. Ascorbic acid tends to melt tooth enamel. Constantly chewing vitamin C tablets is harmful to your teeth. If you must chew, cleanse your mouth immediately afterward.

Do gums vary in color?

Gums have the same origins as skin and pigmentation varies with the color of the skin.

Should you use toothpicks?

Only the kind that don't break or splinter (see Chapter 3). Dental floss is much better and safer.

Should you brush your tongue?

Certainly! It is an important finishing touch to your regular oral hygiene care.

What is the prime cause of tooth loss after age 35?

Periodontal disease. It causes a far greater loss than tooth decay.

What should I do if my gums bleed?

Increasing the length and frequency of brushing your gums and teeth, together with regular professional scaling and cleaning, will control most gum bleeding.

Can I stop my gums from receding?

You can minimize gum recession by using a medium or soft toothbrush and proper brushing techniques with regular oral prophylaxis. Make sure your dentist checks for correct bite.

Can drugs harm your mouth?

Yes. Taking certain drugs (such as Dilantin, used to control epilepsy) may cause change, irritation and inflammation in your gums and may cause tooth decay. Never put an aspirin on a tooth to alleviate a toothache—it burns the gingiva.

Can I readily see the plaque on my teeth?

If you scrape around the neck of a tooth with your fingernail and find a deposit, you can be sure plaque is on the tooth. A disclosing tablet will show it up even better.

Will it hurt to crack a walnut with my teeth?

Yes. While teeth are strong, they also are brittle. It is easy to fracture a tooth.

Is chewing gum harmful?

Yes and no. If you keep popping sugared gum into your mouth all day, that's bad. Sugarless gum is safer. But constantly chewing any gum will wear down your teeth.

What kind of toothbrush should I buy?

Buy a straight-handled brush with rounded, soft to medium-soft bristles, with four rows. Select the size that comfortably fits your mouth. Hard bristles wear down teeth and can injure gums.

How often should I buy a new toothbrush?

If you buy three or four toothbrushes and rotate them, each

will last longer than using only one brush. As soon as the bristles seem to bend, get a new brush. Rinsing with hot water will shorten the life of a toothbrush.

Which is better—a toothbrush with nylon or natural bristles?

Either type is acceptable.

Is it okay to use someone else's toothbrush?

If there is no other toothbrush handy, it's better than not brushing at all.

What can I do when I'm away from home without a toothbrush?

Rinse very vigorously after eating. Warm water will be more effective than cold.

Why do we have so many cavities when less sophisticated civilizations are practically cavity-free?

Most of these civilizations consume more detergent food products and little or no refined sugar.

Is it better to use dental tape than dental floss?

Both work well. However, the wider tape seems to clean the teeth surfaces more efficiently.

Why does a dentist want bitewing x rays so often?

Bitewing x rays aid in early detection of small cavities between teeth.

Can one dentist treat a family of two adults, one senior citizen and two children?

Of course. Especially if the dentist is a general practitioner.

How can I be sure my dental bill is fair?

Dental fees for a specific service should fall within the customary range for your locality. Time, care, difficulty of the case, the dentist's background and training also are factors.

Can I get good treatment in a dental school clinic?

Clinic patients receive excellent care, supervised by competent, experienced teachers. The dental work is of superior quality, although more time is required. The costs are much lower than those of practicing dentists.

Must I be poor to go to a dental school clinic?

No, you can drive up in your chauffeur-driven limousine.

What can I do if a filling falls out on a Sunday?

If you're in pain, try to contact your dentist at home or phone the local dental society for a referral. If it's a gold inlay, by all means save it, as it may be used again. You can also pack the cavity with sterile cotton to relieve pain and keep it clean.

What can I do if I get a toothache at midnight?

Take aspirin or apply oil of cloves to the hurting tooth. Call your dentist in the morning.

Do you get good dental care when you're in the hospital?

Not always. Bring your dental kit with you. If, temporarily, you can't take care of your teeth, ask the nurse to brush for you.

Are x rays dangerous?

Not if the x-ray equipment has been recently checked and certified to be in good order, and if a lead apron covers you from chin to thigh.

What's the best filling I can have?

Gold wherever it is not obvious and the cavity is extensive. Otherwise, amalgam or new composite material.

Why do some individuals need a local anesthetic and others don't?

The younger we are, the larger and more sensitive the tooth's pulp. As we grow older, the pulp gets smaller and there is less sensation.

How much time can modern equipment save you and the dentist when putting in an average filling?

Thirty to fifty percent time—not to mention added comfort.

If I'm always getting food between my teeth, what should I do?

Food impaction is due to improper contacts between teeth. New and properly contoured restorations with tighter contacts are needed.

Do only older people get gumline cavities?

No, anybody can get them.

Receding gums make me look older. What can I do about it?

You may have crowns put on the teeth that show. The crowns will cover the recession, fit snugly up to your gumline and give a younger appearance.

What is bruxism?

Bruxism is the nervous habit of gnashing teeth at night and sometimes under stress during the day. Bruxists clench their jaws and grind so vigorously that they may wear teeth down to the pulp. Severe headaches and facial pain can result.

Can I catch oral diseases by eating in restaurants?

Rarely.

What is gingivoplasty?

Actually it is plastic surgery, involving reshaping and recontouring the gums after periodontal treatment. It helps bring back satisfactory shape.

Has the grafting of gum tissue been successful?

Yes, it has proved successful in repairing defects in gums and it improves appearance.

Has bone graft in dental cases been equally effective?

It has met with varying degrees of success, depending on the area involved.

How can I tell if I'm grinding my teeth while asleep?

Most people who grind their teeth are aware of it, although they don't remember exactly when they were grinding. The abrasion on their teeth is evident.

Does snoring harm your teeth?

Yes. Snoring causes the mouth to dry up. Older porcelain fillings also dry, tend to loosen, and are soon brushed away.

If loose teeth are splintered, how long will they last?

If you get immediate attention for them, they should last a number of additional years, so long as you take good care of them.

When should I go to a periodontist?

When you have symptoms of periodontal disease or when your dentist suggests it.

Should I keep a record of my dental work?

An excellent idea! And keep a record of all dental work for the whole family. In case you move or change dentists, you can explain what treatment was given and when.

Why does a tooth turn dark after root canal treatment?

This is due to the decomposition of pulp tissues and transformation of iron in red blood cells into salts of different colors (red, brown and black). These iron salts penetrate into the tooth, discoloring it.

Is smoking bad for your mouth?

Yes. We see premalignant lesions in patients' mouths all too often. And it doesn't seem to make much difference whether you smoke cigarettes, a pipe or cigars.

Is alcohol harmful?

Strong alcoholic drinks tend to dry and burn the mucous membranes in your mouth. Cells in the mouth may die. Heavy drinking is harmful.

Are fever blisters on the lips the same as canker sores inside the mouth?

They both present many common features and each is caused by the herpes simplex virus.

Can you contract gonorrhea through the mouth?

Yes, if the oral tissues come into direct contact with infected genitalia.

Why is it so difficult to extract an impacted wisdom tooth?

Because it is surrounded by bone and may have several crooked roots.

How long should a fixed bridge last?

From 15 to 25 years, if it's a good bridge.

What are "soft" teeth?

Although some people claim they've inherited "soft" teeth, clinically there is no such thing, except for some specific diseases. What we may inherit is a food pattern, including too many starches and sweets which destroy tooth enamel.

Is it dangerous to chew on a bone?

Yes, if you chew down too hard. Go slowly, take it easy and be careful with teeth that have older fillings or caps.

I have a front tooth that protrudes. Can I push it back in place?

In some cases, gently pressing a finger against a tooth for several hours a day will help. But you should be supervised by a dentist.

At what age should I take my child to the dentist?

Regular visits should begin when most of the baby teeth have erupted—usually about age 2. At this young age, visits to the dental office will be a pleasant experience, since no major work should be required if you're taking good care of the young mouth.

Why is a child better off with a pedodontist?

A pedodontist is trained to handle children psychologically and his office is geared to care for the little ones.

How can I stop my children from eating junk food?

Don't have any in the house. Serve only wholesome, nutritious meals, have fresh fruit around and hide the sugar bowl.

How often should a child have a dental checkup?

At least every 6 months.

Is nail biting bad for your teeth?

It's bad for both teeth and nails. It wears down teeth, nails and causes raw swollen cuticles. Whistle instead.

Should I brush my dog's teeth?

Certainly, if he's agreeable. Teeth should also be cleaned and scaled by the veterinarian at periodic intervals—more frequently as your pet gets older. Tough "chew food" and rawhide chewies will help keep his teeth free of plaque and tartar.

What causes sore spots under my dentures?

The cause is abnormal pressure. The remedy is to give your gums a rest. Remove the dentures most of the time and rinse the mouth often with warm saltwater. Do not file down your dentures. Have the dentist adjust them.

If a tooth gets knocked out, what should I do?

Grab it and put it back in its own socket, if possible. If not, place it under your tongue. Get to a dentist *at once!* He may be able to insert the tooth back in its socket.

If I have root canal treatment, will my tooth still last as long as other teeth?

Yes, provided you are in good health and the fibers supporting the teeth are also healthy. Most root canals should be protected from fracture by a dowel and crown.

Isn't it better to just buy dentures than to spend so much time and money on saving your teeth?

No, false teeth cannot match the comfort and efficiency of natural teeth.

Do toothpastes made for sensitive teeth really help?

These toothpastes seem to help alleviate sensitivity in some cases.

What about toothpastes that claim to whiten your teeth?

Proceed with caution. Such toothpastes usually contain bleaching chemicals and/or coarse abrasive powder.

Is it okay to use salt and lemon juice to remove brown stains from my teeth?

It is effective, but dangerous. Salt is abrasive. Lemon is acid. As you remove the stain, you remove tooth enamel.

Can a dentist bleach my teeth?

Yes. Some discolored teeth can be bleached successfully.

Can my teeth be stained by coffee, tea, iron or potassium in liquid form?

Yes.

I hate to wear a removable partial denture. Can I have a fixed bridge made with an implant?

Sufficient jawbone is needed to support an implant. An implantologist can examine you and advise whether or not your jawbone can receive an implant.

Is it all right to "gum" your food without any teeth at all?

No! Food must be chewed. If you're financially strapped, why not try to locate a dental school or a community clinic where you can get excellent, inexpensive dentures.

How long will good dental plates last?

If you're careful, your dentures should last 6 or 7 years with two or three relinings during that time. It's wise to keep an extra set in case of emergency.

When a tooth is knocked out and quickly replaced, how long will the tooth remain in its socket?

If replanted *immediately,* its chances of lasting are good. There is one case where two replanted teeth have continued to function for 42 years.

GLOSSARY

Abrasion: Grinding or wearing away of tooth structure by mastication, incorrect brushing methods, bruxism, or other damage.

Abscess: Localized pus in a cavity due to disintegration of tissue.

Abutment teeth: Teeth used to support a bridge or partial denture.

Alveolar process: The part of the jawbone where roots of teeth are embedded.

Alveolar socket: The cavity in the alveolar process wherein roots of teeth are embedded.

Apex: Tip of the tooth's root.

Bruxism: Grinding teeth, especially during sleep.

Calcification: Hardening of organic tissue by a deposit of calcium or mineral salts within its substance.

Canker: A shallow ulcer in the mouth or on the lip.

Caries: Tooth decay.

Cast: A reproduction of the dental arch or part of it, made by pouring a mix of plaster or artificial stone into an impression.

Cavity: A hole in a tooth caused by decay.

Cervix: A narrow region around the area of the tooth where crown and root meet.

Compound cavity: A cavity that extends onto more than one surface of the tooth.

Crown: The part of the tooth visible above the gumline or an artificial substitute.

Cusp: A rounded protuberance on or near the chewing surface of a tooth.

Dentin: The substance that makes up the bulk of a tooth, under the enamel.

Dentition: Character of the teeth, as determined by their form and arrangement; also, the development and cutting of teeth.

Diastema: A space between teeth.

Disclosing solution: A liquid that stains plaque on teeth so it can easily be seen and removed.

Enamel: The substance that covers the normally exposed part of the crown.

Endodontics: Dental specialty dealing with diseases and treatment of the dental pulp.

Erosion: The loss of tooth structure, mostly on the facial surfaces of teeth.

Exfoliation: The falling out of teeth.

Facial: Outer surfaces of teeth.

Fissure: A fault in the enamel

Gingiva: A mucous membrane covering the alveolar process and encircling necks of the teeth.

Gingival margin: The gumline, or gum margin.

Gingivectomy: Cutting away some of the gum tissue or a lesion of the gum.

Gingivoplasty: Surgical reshaping and recontouring of gum tissue.

Impacted tooth: A tooth lying in the jawbone in such a manner that it cannot erupt.

Incisal edges: The cutting edges of front teeth.

Inlay: A restoration prepared outside the mouth and cemented into a prepared cavity.

Interproximal space: The space between contacting or adjoining teeth just below the contact area.

Labial: The facial surface of a front tooth.

Lateral: Front tooth adjacent to central incisors.

Lingual: The sides of teeth nearest the tongue.

Malocclusion: Any deviation from normal occlusion, due to teeth that are out of line, causing an improper relationship of the jaws.

Mottling: Discoloration of teeth due to excessive fluoride.

Mucosa: Mucous membranes of the mouth.

Mucous membranes: The linings in canals and cavities of the body.

Occlusion: The relation of the upper and lower teeth and jaws.

Oral pathology: A branch of pathology concerned with the oral cavity and surrounding tissues.

Oral surgery: A surgical specialty relating to the oral cavity.

Orthodontics: A specialty concerned with irregularities of the teeth and their correction.

Pathology: The branch of medical science that deals with the nature of diseases and the structural and functional changes produced by them.

Pedodontics: A children's dental specialty, concerned with normal care and preventing, intercepting and correcting some problems of occlusion.

Periodontal tissues: Tissues that surround and support the roots of the teeth.

Periodontics: The specialty concerned with prevention, examination, diagnosis and treatment of periodontal diseases.

Periodontium: The tissues that help support the teeth, including the gums, the cementum, the periodontal ligament, the alveolar process and supporting bone.

Plaque: A sticky, gelatinlike deposit of material on the surface of a tooth, where bacteria collect and cause tooth decay and gum disease.

Prosthetics: The art and science of supplying, fitting and servicing artificial replacements for missing parts of the body.

Public health: A specialty of dentistry concerned with helping a population group, rather than private patients.

Pulp: Soft vital tissue at the center of the tooth. It forms dentin and maintains the vitality of the tooth.

Pulp cavity: The space in the center of the tooth bounded by the dentin, containing the dental pulp.

Resorption: Gradual removal or destruction of tissues, especially bone.

Restoration: Replacement of a missing tooth structure with a dental material.

Restorative dentistry: Reparative dentistry, involving the replacement of missing teeth, rebuilding, repairing or reforming teeth or portions of teeth.

Root canal therapy: Removal of pulp from the root canal; cleansing, shaping, sterilizing and filling the canal.

Saliva ejector: An aparatus for the removal of saliva and water from the mouth during dental treatment.

Simple cavity: A cavity on only one surface of a tooth.

Supernumerary: An extra tooth.

Tissue: Similar cells united in a particular function.

Topical: Local, pertaining to a special surface or spot.

Toxic: Pertaining to, due to, or of the nature of a poison.

Ultrasonic: Term describing mechanical vibrations beyond the range audible to the human ear, usually above 20,000 vibrations per second.

Undercut: Cutting cavity walls wider at the bottom so that a restoration will not come out.

Virus: Latin word meaning poison. One of a group of widely different agents that infect animals, plants, insects, bacteria and fungi. Viruses are intracellular parasites.

Wisdom tooth: A third molar.

SUGGESTED READING

Accredited Dental Schools. *The Journal of the American Dental Association:* July 1977, pp. 123–125.

Boucher, Carl O. Hickey, Judson C., and Zarb, George A. *Prosthodontic Treatment for Edentulous Patients,* seventh edition. St. Louis: C. V. Mosby, 1975.

Coady, J. M. Future Trends in Dental Education, *Journal of the American College of Dentists:* April 1975, pp. 82–97.

Cohen, S. and Burns, R. C. *Pathways of the Pulp.* St. Louis: C. V. Mosby, 1976.

Craig, G. G., and Dunn, G. R. *A Guide to the Practice of Preventive Dentistry.* Dental Health Education and Research Foundation, The University of Sydney, 1971.

Dental Education. *The Journal of the American Dental Association:* May 1976, pp. 880–883.

Dubner, R. Efficacy and Possible Mechanisms of Action of Acupuncture Anesthesia: Observations Based on a Visit to the People's Republic of China. *The Journal of the American Dental Association:* February 1976, pp. 418–427.

Fechtner, J. L., and Mallin, R. J. 15 Years of Preventive

Dentistry in Private Practice. *The Journal of the American Dental Association:* April 1972, pp. 817–823.

Fluoridation Facts. American Dental Association Educational Booklet, 1974.

French, M. Perspective on Prevention. *Journal of the American College of Dentists:* April 1975, pp. 98–106.

Glickman, Irving. *Clinical Periodontology: Recognition, Diagnosis and Treatment of Periodontal Disease in the Practice of General Dentistry,* fourth edition. Philadelphia: W. B. Saunders, 1972.

Glickman, Irving, *et al. Periodontal Disease: Clinical, Radiographic and Histopathologic Features.* Philadelphia: W. B. Saunders, 1974.

Goldman, *et al. Current Therapy in Dentistry,* Vol. 5. St. Louis: C. V. Mosby, 1974.

Goldman, Henry M., and Cohen, D. Walter. *Periodontal Therapy,* fifth edition. St. Louis: C. V. Mosby, 1973.

Judy, K. W. M., and Weiss, C. M., editors. *The International Journal of Oral Implantology:* Vol. 1, No. 1; October 1976.

Laws, P. W. *Medical and Dental X-rays.* Washington, DC: Public Citizen Health Research Group, 1975.

McDonald, R. E. *Dentistry for the Child and Adolescent,* second edition. St. Louis: C. V. Mosby, 1974.

McGuire, T. *The Tooth Trip.* New York: Random House, 1972.

Moss, S. J., *et al. Preventive Dentistry.* New York: Medocom, Inc., 1972.

Park, Virginia R., *et al. A Textbook for Dental Assistants.* Philadelphia: W. B. Saunders, 1975.

Petersen, S. *Comprehensive Review for Dental Hygienists,* second edition. St. Louis: C. V. Mosby, 1969.

Stoll, F. A., and Catherman, J. L. *Dental Health Education,* fourth edition. Philadelphia: Lea & Febiger, 1972.

Developing a Plaque Control Program. University of California School of Dentistry, Berkeley, California; Praxis Publishing Co., 1972.

Wilkins, E. M. *Clinical Practice of the Dental Hygienist,* third edition. Philadelphia: Lea & Febiger, 1973.

INDEX